52 Juice & Smoothie Recipes

One for each week of the year!

By

Andy Williams, Ph.D.

Table of Contents

Disclaimer

The author and publisher of this eBook and the accompanying materials have used their best efforts in preparing this eBook. The author and publisher make no representation or warranties with respect to the accuracy, applicability, fitness, or completeness of the contents of this eBook. The information contained in this eBook is strictly for educational purposes. Therefore, if you wish to apply ideas contained in this eBook, you are taking full responsibility for your actions. The information and advice in this book is not medical advice. If you have medical problems, consult your physician.

The author and publisher disclaim any warranties (express or implied), merchantability, or fitness for any particular purpose. The author and publisher shall in no event be held liable to any party for any direct, indirect, punitive, special, incidental or other consequential damages arising directly or indirectly from any use of this material, which is provided "as is", and without warranties.

The author and publisher do not warrant the performance, effectiveness or applicability of any sites listed or linked to in this eBook.

All links are for information purposes only and are not warranted for content, accuracy or any other implied or explicit purpose.

Introduction

What better way to get your daily intake of fruit & vegetables, than by creating delicious juices and smoothies?

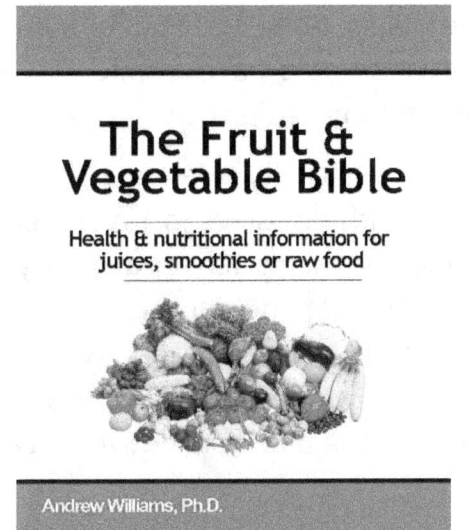

The Fruit & Vegetable Bible

Health & nutritional information for juices, smoothies or raw food

Andrew Williams, Ph.D.

This book includes 52 recipes, one for each week of the year for you to try. Each one uses a different main ingredient, meaning you never get bored, but always get drinks packed with nutrition and variety.

One thing you won't find in this book is large, colourful pictures of the drinks. Photos just take more downloading, meaning I have to charge more for the book. If you want to see what a drink looks like, make it!

If you want to try these recipes, but don't have a juicer or blender, why not pop over to my site at http://JuicingTheRainbow.com and drop me an email. I'll be only too happy to help you find the perfect machine(s) for your requirements (and budget).

If you would like more information on these 52 fruit, vegetables and herbs, check out my Fruit & Vegetable Bible.

This recipe book was written as a companion to that book. The Fruit & Vegetable Bible is available on Amazon in Kindle format and as a paperback. Search Amazon for it by name, or by its ASIN number, which is B00JVPLDV0.

OK, without further ado, let's get on with the recipes.

Alfalfa Sprouts: Very Berry Sprouted Smoothie

Summary: alfalfa sprouts are a product of alfalfa seeds. The tiny sprouts are thread-like in structure with green tops. The seeds can be cultivated anywhere on the planet irrespective of climate or temperature. The highly nutritive sprouts have a mild taste making them the ideal addition to any smoothie recipe.

Belonging to the pea family, alfalfa is actually a legume. They can easily be harvested for home smoothie recipes in just seven days and while adding excessive amounts might deliver a 'grassy' taste to the drink, just a small quantity of the sprouts has the ability to boost the nutritive value of the drink significantly. The year-round availability makes them a convenient and inexpensive smoothie ingredient which rejuvenates the body and delivers age defying nutrients.

Very Berry Sprouted Smoothie Recipe

- ¼ Cup Alfalfa Sprouts
- 1 Stalks Organic Celery
- ½ Banana
- ½ cup Frozen Mixed Berries
- ½ Cup Fresh Orange Juice

Place all ingredients in a blender and blend thoroughly.

Add-ons

- ¼ inch fresh ginger, minced
- ½ cup pineapple
- ½ cup baby spinach

Nutritional Information

Alfalfa sprouts have an abundance of nutrients like calcium, manganese, folic acid, magnesium, phosphorous, molybdenum, silicon, potassium, zinc and sodium. Additionally it provides a wide array of vitamins like vitamin A in the form of beta carotene, B6, B12, C, D, E as well as K.

Alfalfa sprouts also contains vital enzymes. Lipase is the tearing enzyme, amylase breaks down starches, coagulase clots blood, emulsin converts carbohydrate compounds to glucose, invertase converts transforms cane sugar to dextrose, peroxidate has an oxidizing effect on the blood, pectinase forms vegetable jelly and protease aids in digesting proteins.

Health benefits of Alfalfa Sprouts

Alfalfa sprouts supply the body with a large array of nutrients that aid in the overall well-being and fitness of the body. They are the greatest source of anti-oxidants among all vegetables and can aid in alleviating many degenerative diseases like osteoporosis, heart disease, and menopausal symptoms to name a few. The anti-inflammatory compounds help those suffering from arthritis. Some studies indicate that the amino-acid known as L-canavanine found in alfalfa sprouts might the natural compound effective against leukemia. Regular use of alfalfa sprouts boosts the immune system. The sprouts are not only gentle but healing as well for patients with ulcers.

Apples: Versatile Apple Juice

Apples are the most commonly cultivated and consumed fruit on the planet, making them easily accessible. Their naturally sweet taste, high nutritive value, and ease of blending with other fruits or vegetables make them the ideal juicing candidate.

Apples are frequently referred to as a "miracle food" due to the exceptionally vital flavonoids, antioxidants and dietary fibre found in the fruit. The nutrient packed juice makes the perfect thirst quencher for children as well as adults

Some precautions that should be considered when juicing include the removal of the apple pips. The pips contain tiny amounts of cyanide and while one would have to consume hugely large amounts of the pips to feel the effects of the poison, it is best to core the apples before juicing. Many people prefer to remove the peels before juicing due to pesticide residue concerns. However, laboratory tests have failed to find any significant deposits after repeated tests, and the apple skin contains a significant amount of the nutrients, which gets discarded unnecessarily if the apple is peeled before juicing.

Versatile Apple Juice Ingredients:

- 4 large apples (preferably of 2 or 3 different varieties for better tasting juice)

Scrub the apples thoroughly, remove the core and cut into pieces that will fit in your juice extractor machine. Many people prefer to combine the apple juice with juice from vegetables like carrots, celery, or cucumber to get the benefits the vegetables have to offer. Combining not only disguises the flavour of the vegetables but it also reduces the natural sweetness of apples.

Add-ons

- Carrots
- Celery
- Pineapple

Nutritional Information

The star nutrients in apples are polyphenols which include flavonols, catechins, anthocyanins, and dozens of others which support good health. Additionally apples are rich in fibre and house an array of vitamins including A, C, E, K, thiamin, riboflavin, folates, and niacin. They also contain sodium, potassium, iron, calcium, magnesium, phosphorus and zinc. Furthermore apples are low in saturated fat, cholesterol and sodium.

Health Benefits of Apples

Apples have elevated levels of the soluble fibre pectin which is useful in removing toxic wastes like lead, aluminum and mercury from the body. It binds with radioactive deposits in the body and eliminates them. The malic and tartaric acids found in the juice slow down the spread of harmful bacteria in the intestines and trigger production of beneficial bacteria. Apple juice lowers cholesterol according to researchers at The Florida State University, and its high mineral content is good for healthy hair, skin and fingernails.

The antioxidant "quercetin" in apple juice reduces cellular death due to inflammation and oxidation of neurons according to University of Quebec researchers. A Cornell University study, published in the Journal of Food and Science has found evidence that apple juice may lower the chances of developing Alzheimer's disease and colon cancer. Another Cornell study found that the phenolic compounds in apples may aid in preventing breast cancer.

Asparagus: Asparagus Divinity

Rich in dietary fibre and packed with vitamins, asparagus is considered to be a delicacy among vegetables. A bit on the pricy side due to the need for hand harvesting, it is easily available all year round, but is best during spring.

Asparagus is more often better recognized for the distinctive smell it produces in urine of individuals who consume it, rather than being prized for the nutrition it offers. The smell is produced when the compound mercaptan is metabolized by the body. The same compound is also responsible for the smell produced by skunks, garlic, onions and rotting eggs. Not everyone consuming asparagus produces the smell and not everyone who produces it, has the ability to smell it. The production and the ability to smell it are related to the genes of individuals.

Asparagus divinity Ingredients:

- 5 spears of asparagus
- 2 large carrots
- 1 small cucumber

Process each ingredient through the juicer. Depending on personal taste strain if needed but remember the more you strain the lesser the fibre content your body gets. If necessary the juice can be further sweetened with a bit of honey or some other sweetener.

Add-ons

- Celery
- Tomato

Nutritional Information

One of the best diet foods, asparagus delivers only 40 calories per cup, no sodium, fat or cholesterol and plenty of fibre. It is a great source of folate, potassium, vitamins A, C and K with a hint of vitamin B. It is one of a limited number of vegetables which actually supplies calcium. It is also a good source of magnesium

Health Benefits of Asaparagus

The prebiotics in asparagus stimulate friendly bacteria in the intestine to grow, which aids digestion and keeps the digestive system in top shape. The potassium in the veggie helps to regulate blood pressure and is accredited with cutting down on fat deposits, while the folic acid reduces the blood homocysteine levels that lessen the risks of heart disease. The Vitamin K found in asparagus is known for carrying out bone formation and repair work.

A specific type of phytochemical found in asparagus endow it with anti-inflammatory properties that are effective in relieving arthritis and rheumatism. The glutathione (an anti-oxidant) in the vegetable is believed to aid in cancer prevention in addition to cataracts and other eye problems. Asparagus is a natural diuretic and when taken in the form of a juice its effect is enhanced, making it a great body detoxifier.

Avocado: Merry Berry Avocado Shake

Despite being a bit fatty, consumed in moderation avocados are good for health. They deliver roughly twenty vitamins and minerals in a single serving.

Also known recognized by the name "alligator pear," the avocado is a prized fruit in terms of the nutritional value it provides. The skin of an avocado is thick and varies in colour from vibrant green to nearly black. Its texture may be smooth or pebbled while the flesh is creamy with a yellowish green colouration. In the middle there is one large pit.

Like bananas, avocados only ripen after the mature fruit is picked from the tree. After removal from the plant, avocados ripen within a few days, leaving only a short duration during which the fruit can be consumed. The mature fruit is rather hard to the touch, however when ripe, the tight skin will yield slightly if squeezed. Research shows that the maximum concentration of nutrients is located just under the skin. This is why it is vital to remove only the minimum amount of skin. To ensure that no nutrients are lost, it is best to peel the avocado like a banana as the skin comes off with ease.

Merry Berry Avocado Shake Ingredients:

- ½ cup peeled and diced avocado
- 1 banana
- ½ cup milk
- 1 cup frozen strawberries
- ¼ cup plain yogurt
- ½ teaspoon cinnamon

Add the milk, yogurt, banana and avocado into a blender and mix until smooth or about thirty seconds. Next add the berries and blend thoroughly. Pour into glasses and sprinkle with cinnamon.

Add-ons

- Blueberries
- Honey

Nutritional Information

A one hundred gram serving of avocado supplies 26% of the daily recommended allowance of vitamin K, 20% folate, 17% vitamin C, 14% vitamin B5 and potassium, 13% vitamin B6, and 10% vitamin E. it also supplies smaller amounts of magnesium, copper, manganese, zinc, iron, phosphorus, vitamin A, B1, B2 and B3. Furthermore, avocados contain very little saturated fat, no cholesterol or sodium.

Health Benefits of Avocado

Avocados offer numerous health benefits. The compound beta-sitosterol, found in ample quantities in avocados has been shown to lower the LDL (bad cholesterol), while increasing HDL (good cholesterol) according one study. Compounds like glutathione, monounsaturated fat and vitamin E in avocados aide in keeping the heart healthy, while phytonutrients like polyphenols and flavonoids are known to deliver anti-inflammatory benefits that help to avert inflammation related disorders like arthritis. The fruit also offers protection against cataracts and age-related macular degeneration and is also known to increase carotenoid absorption by as much as five times. The soluble fiber helps to maintain steady blood sugar levels.

Basil: Basil Berry Delight

Basil is a very fragrant herb that has traditionally been used as a seasoning and garnish in cooking. Recently it has become an important ingredient in juicing recipes due to the numerous health benefits it offers. While the leaves are the most commonly used part of the plant, its seeds, flowers and stem are equally nutritious.

Basil leaves are among the oldest known herbs with aromatic qualities as well as medicinal worth. There are approximately 35 basil species found growing around the world. They differ from each other in structure and the essential oils found in them. The sweet basil and Holy Basil are the most commonly grown varieties. Holy Basil is traditionally employed in Indian Ayurveda medicine and is referred to in ancient Hindu texts.

The taste and aroma of the herb is due to the oils found in the leaves, roots, stem and seeds of the plant. The varying compositions of the oils give rise to the different species with varying aromas. Sweet basil produces a clove like scent because of the eugenol present in the species. Egenol is also found in cloves. Lemon basil house citral and imonene giving rise to citrus smell while Licorice Basil contains anethole giving it anise smell.

Basil Berry Delight Ingredients:

- Handful of basil leaves
- 5 whole strawberries
- 1 cup water
- Honey to taste

Add-ons

- Pineapple
- Mango

- Carrots

Nutritional Information

Basil leaves offer an abundant supply of vitamin A and K. Additionally they are a good source of Vitamin C, B6, Folat, Niacin and Vitamin E. In the mineral department they provide manganese, calcium, copper, potassium, iron, magnesium, and zinc. They also provide a hefty amount of dietary fibers, roughly 25% of the dried herb by weight is fiber. Basil contains the water-soluble flavonoids orientin and vicenin. The seeds contain carbohydrates minerals and vitamins.

Health Benefits of Basil Leaves

In Ayurveda medicine basil leaves are thought to be the remedy for all ailments. People are encouraged to chew the fresh leaves to gain maximum health benefits. Numerous ayurvedic products such as tulsi powder, tea, skin cream and capsules are commonly available.

A brew of green tulsi leaves with some ginger is believed to prevent malaria and dengue fever. Leaves boiled with cardamom powder, and honey is an aide for bringing down fever. The leaves also have anti-viral and microbial properties that help to bring down fever and control growth of virus and bacteria. Fungal infections can be treated with applying crushed leaves to the infected region. Oils in the herb are a natural insect repellant and insecticide.

Some powerful components like camphene, eugenol and vitamin C with decongesting properties that help to cure lung damage caused tuberculosis. Tulsi leaves are believed to be a natural cure of Croup, an ailment in which larynx is blocked.

Beets: Beet & Greens Juice

Beets are the source of betanin and vulgaxanthin, two of the best-studied betalains. Both of these nutrients provide antioxidant, anti-inflammatory, and detoxification properties. While betalains can be found in other foods, beets have the highest concentration of these highly valuable nutrients.

Beet juice provides some very powerful benefits and only a small quantity, one to two ounces a week, is sufficient to attain them. It is best to juice the whole beet inclusive of roots, stems and greens as most of the minerals and vitamins are stored in the greens. In fact beet greens contain more iron than spinach and offer greater nutritional value on the whole than the beetroot on its own. The juice may be consumed on its own or combined with other fruits and vegetables to produce a healthy refreshing drink.

Beets are best when consumed raw as the most beneficial compounds like betalains are lost during cooking. Additionally oxalic acid, found mostly in high levels in beet greens is harmful when cooked, but when used in moderation in the raw form, it is beneficial. Individuals who have kidney stones or are on a restricted oxalate diet should use Beet Greens Juice sparingly. Consumption of beet juice may turn urine and stool red. This is perfectly normal and not a cause for alarm; an estimated ten to fifteen percent of U.S adults experience this phenomenon.

Beet & Greens Juice Ingredients:

- 1 beet with greens
- 1 spear celery
- 1 medium sized green apple
- ½ lemon juice

Thoroughly wash all produce with cold water and slice the beets, greens, celery and the apple into sizes that will fit the juicer with ease. After juicing add the juice of half a lemon, chill and enjoy.

Add-ons

- Carrot
- Cucumber
- pineapple

Nutritional Information

Juice of beets and greens is an outstanding source of vitamin C, betaine, and salicylic acid. It is also a good source of vitamin A (beta-carotene), calcium, iron, potassium, sulfur, and choline. Beet juice also supplies elevated amounts of minerals that make liver and gall bladder stronger and provide the building blocks for cells.

Health Benefits Beet Juice

The oxalic acid in raw beet juice is known to dissolve inorganic (bad) calcium. Calcium deposits are a major cause of chronic diseases like arthritis, cancer, heart disease, eye problems, and arteriosclerosis. This explains why beet juice is linked with providing relief from symptoms related to these diseases.

Beet juice provides 27% of the recommended daily allowance of folic acid which is known to prevent birth defects. The carotenoids, lutein and zeaxanthin in beet juice are very beneficial to eye health and they are destroyed if cooked. The betaine protects liver and the bile ducts. Beet juice is very good at healing gout, it lowers homocysteine, serum cholesterol, and normalize blood pressure and elevates the stomach acid production.

Blackberries: Blackberry-Green Smoothie

Blackberries are loaded with powerful antioxidants responsible for fighting free radicals and warding off some of the most common modern diseases. Juicing the berries maintains all these benefits.

Blackberries are a highly perishable food that has to be used soon after purchase. The good thing about blackberries is that freezing gives them a longer life without any significant loss in nutrients. Frozen berries can be used in smoothies, juices and cooked preparations. While consumers tend to prefer the newer varieties without the seeds, blackberry seeds contain potent nutrients like omega-3 and 6 fatty acids, protein, and carotenoids to name a few. Making smoothies or juicing blackberries means you don't have to deal with the seeds as they get crushed and still provide all the benefits.

Blackberry-Green Smoothie Ingredients:

- 1 cup blackberries
- ½ cup low-fat yoghurt
- 2 cups fresh spinach leaves
- ½ cup ice cubes

Add all ingredients into a high power blender. Blend on high speed for about 15 seconds, or until a creamy texture is attained! Serve immediately.

Add-ons

- Lemon
- Cabbage
- Celery

Nutritional Information

A one cup serving of blackberries delivers only 62 calories, while supplying two grams of protein, fourteen grams of carbohydrates, one gram of fat, and eight grams of dietary fibre. This satisfies 32% of the day's fibre needs. The same serving size also provides 50% vitamin C, 36% vitamin K, 9% of folate, 7% magnesium and potassium, 6% of vitamins A and E, and 5% of the daily needs of iron, niacin and zinc.

Blackberries contain elevated amounts of gallic acid, ellagic acid and rutin which are recognized to be chemo-preventive, with anti-viral and anti-bacterial characteristics. They also have the greatest antioxidant values.

Health Benefits of Blackberries

A December 2006 study published in the "Journal of Agriculture and Food Chemistry" found that blackberry extracts avert the growth of cancer cell in tests carried out in laboratories. The greater the quantities of berries consumed, the higher the degree of protection.

The fibre along with minerals, phytochemicals found in blackberries might aid in lowering the risk of heart disease according to 2010 article published in "Nutrition Reviews". The pathways employed in lowering these risks include reduction in inflammation and oxidative stress by increasing antioxidants in the blood, and lowering of cholesterol due to the presence of anthocyanins, the phytochemicals responsible for giving blackberries their dark colour.

Consumption of blackberries may also aid in forestalling age related cognitive function decline. A 2009 study published in "Nutritional Neuroscience" found that rats supplemented with a two percent blackberry diet performed better on short-term memory tests as compared to those not given the supplement.

Blueberries: Frozen Blueberry Charm

Consuming two cups of blueberries surpasses the benefits of all other types of berries combined. When combined with other healthy vegetables like cabbage, spinach or kale they make for great tasting healthy drinks that even children enjoy.

Blueberries are typically enjoyed in jams, jellies, baked goods or cheesecakes, but they are great for eating out of hand or juicing also. Being dark in color and naturally very sweet means they can hide flavours of some healthy vegetables, making them great candidates of smoothies or juicing.

Due to their low vitamin C content compared to other fruits, blueberries were not given due attention for the longest time. Later discoveries showed that blueberries are a super-food like none other, due to their phytonutrients and antioxidant content. While a delicate fruit, blueberries can be frozen when in season for greater convenience, without causing any damage to their nutritional content.

Frozen Blueberry Charm Ingredients

- 1 Cup Skim Milk
- 1 Cup Yogurt
- 1 Cup Blueberries
- 1 Cup Ice-cubes
- 1 teaspoon sweetener of choice

Place all ingredients in a blender and mix for ten to twenty seconds depending on how smooth you like your drink.

Add-ons

- Honey

- Celery

Nutritional Information

One cup of blueberries contains only 84 calories, no fat, cholesterol or sodium. It also supplies one gram of protein and two grams of dietary fibre making them a very healthy food. Consuming blueberries is a good way to enhance your vitamin intake. They provide vitamins A, C, E and K. They are also a source of essential minerals like manganese, and small amounts of iron, potassium and copper. The deep purple of blueberries is due to the phytonutrient anthocyanin, which is also now associated with many health benefits in humans.

Health Benefits of Blueberries

When compared to forty other fruits and vegetables blueberries ranked at the top in terms of antioxidant activity. Antioxidants strengthen the immune system by neutralizing the free radicals in the body. Most of this antioxidant power is due to the anthocyanins in blueberries.

The compound pterostilbene in blueberries is accredited with reducing the accumulation of "bad". The compound holds the potential to be developed into a cholesterol lowering nutraceutical. It will be especially useful for individuals who do not respond well to conventional drugs.

Researchers at the Rutgers University in New Jersey have discovered a compound in blueberries that inhibits bacteria from sticking to urinary tract cells and cut down on urinary tract infections. Consumption of blueberries is also found to be beneficial in slowing down age-related loss of mental capacity and improved eyesight.

Broccoli: Minty Broccoli Mix

Broccoli is packed with nutrients, phytonutrients and anti-oxidants. It is also highly valued for its abundance of anti-viral, anti-ulcer and anti-cancer activities, in addition to its natural ability to cleanse the liver. This easily available vegetable is packed with nutrients and offers an inexpensive to remain healthy.

A lot of people just find the idea of consuming green juices highly disagreeable due to either the colour or taste. What they don't realize is that in direct comparison with milk, it has almost the same amount of calcium and more protein minus the lactose and toxins found in milk. This makes consumption of broccoli juice almost a must.

To deal with the taste and colour, it is possible to combine broccoli juice with other fruits or vegetables. For example adding carrots or strawberries gives the juice a beautiful pink/orange tint which is pleasing to the eye and taste buds. An added benefit is that not only do you get the goodness of broccoli but you also get the benefits carrots and strawberries have to offer, like vitamin C, beta-carotene and ellagic acid. Herbs can also be added to further enhance the flavour and aroma of the drink.

Minty Broccoli Mix Ingredients:

- 3 stalks of broccoli
- 2 medium sized apples
- A healthy helping of fresh mint

Wash everything thoroughly, remove and discard any rotting or over-ripe portions. Cut into pieces small enough to fit your juicer and juice a few pieces at a time.

Add-ons

- Ginger
- Pineapple

Nutritional Information

Broccoli is low in calories and yet loaded with some unique disease fighting ingredients. It contains important anti-oxidants like quercetin, beta-carotene, glutathione, indoles, vitamin C, lutein, sulphoraphane and glucarate. Broccoli is also very good in the vitamin and mineral department. It is an exceptionally rich source of vitamins A, C, K, B6, and E in addition to calcium, folate, potassium, magnesium and phosphorus.

Health Benefits of Broccoli

Broccoli juice helps to prevent skin cancer because it contains compounds that elevate the production of protective enzymes that work against different facets of ultraviolet damage by working from inside the cell. The gluocraphanin works to decrease blood pressure and damaging inflammation in the arteries and the heart. The sulforaphane helps to protect the body against the bacteria responsible for causing gastrointestinal problems, thus averting stomach ulcers and bloating. The calcium in broccoli juice works to maintain bone health and burn fat. It also reduces production of cortisol, a stress hormone linked with stomach fat.

Brussel Sprouts: Sunshine Orange & Brussels Sprout Juice

Brussels sprouts, like other members of the same family are known for their immunity-promoting and anti-cancer properties. Drinking the juice ensures that the maximum amount of nutrients are absorbed by the body. The juice is best consumed as soon as possible after extraction as allowing it to sit in the air will deplete some of the health building components.

What was once thought to be a staple to be consumed during the Christmas holidays is now a high-end juice sold at an exclusive store in the United Kingdom. The makers of the juice believe it is the perfect way to enjoy this super food and take advantage of all its nutrients.

The hard-core juicers who prefer the do it yourself method, Brussels sprouts can be juiced in combination with spinach and kale or consumed on its own. Others may find the taste to be a bit overpowering, so adding a pear, berries or apples can make it more palatable. Use only about ¼ cup of Brussels sprout juice and top off the remaining with fruits of choice.

Sunshine Orange Brussels Sprout Juice Ingredients:

- 2 carrots
- 2 apples
- 2 broccoli spears

Add-ons

- Ginger
- Lemon
- strawberries

Nutritional Information

Brussels sprouts are loaded with vitamins A, C, E, B6, and K. This miniature cabbage also supplies significant amounts of minerals which include manganese, potassium, iron, calcium, magnesium, phosphorus, molybdenum, in addition to omega-3 fatty acids and protein. The real value of this vegetable is in its disease combating phytochemicals that include coumarins, dithiolthiones, glucosinolates, indoles, isothiocynates phenols and sulforaphane.

Health Benefits of Brussels Sprout

The phytonutrients contained in Brussels sprouts promote the body's defense systems. They deactivate chemicals responsible for causing cancer and promote enzymes that detoxify the body. Brussels sprouts keep DNA healthy. DNA holds center stage in cell division, and if it gets damaged, cells start to duplicate much faster than normal, this can cause cancerous tumors to form. A number of studies support the Brussels sprouts ability to protect DNA, thereby lower the risks of cancers especially prostrate, bladder, and breast.

The high levels of vitamin C in Brussels Sprouts aid in averting heart disease, and strengthen the immune system. It also fights eye conditions related to eyes including macular degeneration and cataracts. The vitamin K in Brussels sprouts is responsible for blood coagulation and maintaining bone health.

The phytonutrient sulforaphane helps to maintain healthy blood vessels and even reverse previous damage. It is also responsible for regulating inflammation which aids in averting diseases like atherosclerosis, and arthritis. Brussels are also accredited with lowering blood pressure further reducing the risks of heart disease. Lastly, Brussels sprouts help to aid weight loss, digestion and maintain blood sugar levels.

Cabbage: Sweet Cabbage Melody

Cabbage belongs to a family that is traditionally known as cruciferous vegetables. The group is known for supplying nutrients across a wide variety of categories and body systems. The easy to grow vegetable that is easily available around the globe all year comes in numerous varieties, with each providing unique health benefits.

It is now known that the different varieties of cabbage, most common among which are green, red, Nappa, savoy and bok choy, house glucosinolates with differing patterns. Hence to attain the broadest benefits, it is best to include and alternate all varieties in your diet. The Harvard School of Public Health confirms that the use of cabbage in the diet on a regular basis may decrease the chances of developing a large variety of chronic diseases.

Cabbage is loaded with cancer fighting properties, but cooking it destroys the special enzymes, especially myrosinase, which provide the vegetable with its healing powers. Drinking cabbage juice as a healing tonic every few days is the best option for obtaining all the benefits it has to offer. Drinking the juice straight might not suite everyone's taste, but can easily be combined with other health promoting juices to produce a mixture of great tasting drinks.

Sweet Cabbage Melody Ingredients:

- One medium apple
- two large carrots
- ½ head of cabbage

Select fresh cabbage and wash thoroughly along with other fruits and vegetables. Cut all the ingredients into a size that will easily fit the juicer and juice away!

Add-ons

- lemon
- celery

Nutritional Information

Cabbage juice is packed with vital nutrients, providing excellent quantities of vitamins C, K, B6, Folate acid, as well as manganese and glucosinolates. If consumed raw it also supplements the diet with great quantities of fibre. Additionally it is a good source of iron, calcium, thiamin, phosphorus, potassium, and magnesium.

Health Benefits of Cabbage

Four of the glucosinolates in cabbage that have gotten special attention include indole-3-carbinol, sulforaphane, di-indolmethane, and isothiocyanates. They are converted into isothiocyanates in the body and trigger the antioxidant defense apparatus which give the vegetable its special detoxifying and anti-cancer abilities. Cabbage also has anti-inflammatory properties, making it a good food for people suffering from inflammation related issues. According to a study by Stanford University cabbage juice is the most effective natural remedy for people with peptic ulcers. Cabbage also linked with possible macular degeneration of the eyes due to age. The lactic acid in cabbage is helpful in providing relief from muscle sores.

Cantaloupe: Tangy Cantaloupe Juice

When people consider healthy fruits, cantaloupe typically does not come to mind. This is unfortunate because the diversity of nutrients provided by a cantaloupe is a major health factor overlooked by most people.

The cantaloupe is recognized by two main elements, its rough netted stone and greenish skin. When ripe, its flesh is juicy and sweet tasting with floral musky aroma. When lightly pressed at the bottom end (opposite the scarred end where it is cut from the stem), it should yield just a little.

Juicing experts recommend that cantaloupe should not be mixed with other types of fruits or vegetables. This is due to the fact that cantaloupes are nutrient rich and provide a large variety of nutrients on their own without adding anything. This does not mean it can't be combined, just that from nutritional standpoint it is not necessary. Furthermore, when juicing cantaloupes the whole fruit, inclusive of rind and seeds can be used. These parts house a wealth of nutrients which are otherwise wasted.

Tangy Cantaloupe Juice Ingredients:

- ½ cantaloupe
- 2 medium sized oranges
- A healthy pinch of cinnamon

Wash the melon and if using the whole fruit, take extra care to scrub away the dust with a brush. Cut into wedges small enough to fit your juicer and juice. Combine with juice of the oranges and a hint of cinnamon to boost metabolism. It is best to consume the juice immediately to gain the maximum benefits.

Add-ons

- Carrots

- Strawberries

Nutritional Information

Cantaloupes are very good suppliers of vitamins A and C, good suppliers of potassium and a number of B vitamins like B1, B3, B6 and folate in addition to vitamin K, and magnesium. When seeds are also juiced a limited amount of omega-3 fats are also supplied.

Cantaloupes contain the carotenoids alpha and beta carotene as well as their derivatives lutein and zeaxanthin along with the flavonoid luteolin. The anti-inflammatory cucurbitacins B and E are also present in the fruit.

Health Benefits of Cantaloupe

Metabolic syndrome is a group of five conditions including elevated sugar levels, blood pressure and triglycerides, excess body fat around the waist and low HDL (good) cholesterol levels that together increase the chances of heart disease, diabetes and stroke. Typically these problems are associated with undesirable inflammation, and stress resulting from lifestyles. Individuals with greater intake of cantaloupes and other fruits have been observed to have decreased risks of metabolic syndrome. This is due to the fact that cantaloupe contains a broad range of antioxidants known to aid in preventing oxidative stress and anti-inflammatory phytonutrients.

Carrot: Zesty Carrot Juice

Carrots are a source of many essential minerals and nutrients. Its rich supply of antioxidants and other nutrient offer cardiovascular benefits along with anti-cancer benefits.

Carrots are a popular root vegetable that is readily available in every corner of the planet. They are easy to grow, resist most pests and diseases and tolerate cold harsh environment fairly well. Initially carrots were available in all colours from purple to white except orange! The Dutch are credited with developing the orange carrot during the Middle Ages.

Their ease of availability, naturally sweet flavour and crunchy texture makes them a favourite with people of all ages. While they provide a wide array of nutrients and health benefits, overconsumption of the carotene they contain cause the skin to attain a slight colouration. However this is unlikely to be achieved with diet alone, usually over ingestion of vitamin A is caused by supplementation. Cutting back on vitamin A intake can reverse the condition and it is not harmful to health.

Zesty Carrot Juice Ingredients:

- 5 large carrots
- 3 centimeter piece of ginger
- ½ teaspoon lemon

Peel the ginger, remove the lemon's rind and meticulously wash the carrots to ensure that all dirt has been removed. It is not necessary to peel the carrots, just chop them into sizes that your juicer can handle with ease. Juice all ingredients and enjoy it chilled. This juice is great for keeping colds at bay.

Add-ons

- cinnamon

Nutritional Information

Most varieties of carrots are roughly 88 per cent water, seven per cent sugar, one per cent protein, fibre, and ash and contain only 0.2 per cent fat. The United States Department of agriculture defies ½ a cup of chopped carrots as one serving, which in addition to water delivers 25 calories, 6 grams of carbohydrates, 3 grams of sugars and 1 gram of protein.

Carrots are an exceptional source of vitamin A, supplying a little over 200 per cent of an adult's daily needs. They also take care of six per cent of an adult's vitamin C needs, 2 per cent calcium and iron needs in a single serving. The orange colour of the vegetable is due to its beta-carotene content. The beta-carotene is absorbed in the intestine and transformed into vitamin A. Carrots also contain vitamins K, and E potassium manganese, folate, magnesium phosphorous and zinc.

Health Benefits of Carrots

The best known health benefit of carrots is good vision due to the high content of beta-carotene, which is known to provide protection against macular degeneration and age related cataracts. What is not common knowledge is the fact that beta-carotene behaves as an antioxidant that reduces cell damage and slows aging of cells. Consumption of carrots has also been linked to reduction of lung, breast, and colon cancer in some studies. The carotenoids alpha-carotene and lutein in carrots aid in lowering heart disease and grated carrots combined with honey make a great mask for glowing skin.

Cauliflower: Quintessential Cauliflower Juice

While cauliflower is the least nutrient rich member of the cruciferous family, its unique blend of anti-cancerous and anti-inflammatory micro-nutrients make it a must have juice. It should be consumed on a rotational basis with other members of the family.

It is a given that cauliflower will not produce a lot of juice. However, its numerous health benefits make it a mandatory addition to your diet. It is usually enjoyed as an addition to juices that are mostly made up of other fruits and vegetables.

The substance purine occurs naturally in cauliflower is broken down into uric acid in the body. Excessive consumption of the juice can lead to elevated uric acid levels in the body and may lead to problems like kidney stones or gout. So it is best to limit cauliflower juice to once or twice a week, where you are able to gain the benefits without the negative side effects.

Quintessential Cauliflower Juice Ingredients:

- 1 large cucumber
- 4 cups chopped cauliflower
- 2 large apples

Wash and cut all ingredients so they are small enough to fit your juicer. Start juicing with cucumber, then add the apples and finish off with the cauliflower. The apples add a nice sweeting to a refreshing drink, but if you find it to be too sweet you can reduce the apple to just one.

Add-ons

- Carrots
- lemon

Nutritional Information

One hundred grams of cauliflower contain absolutely no cholesterol, hardly any fats, and five grams of carbohydrates and almost two grams of protein. Additionally it supplies 80% of the daily requirement of vitamin C, 10% of vitamin B6, 8% potassium, 3% magnesium and 2% of iron and calcium and 1% sodium. It also supplies some very vital micronutrients like sulforaphane, indole-3-carbinol and Di-indolyl-methane.

Health Benefits of Cauliflower

The sulforaphane is a sulfur compound known for its ability to kill cancer stem cells and slowing tumor growth. Research indicates that combining cauliflower with curcumin, the active ingredient in turmeric can might prevent and treat prostate cancer. Sulforaphane also improves kidney and blood function. The Indoles have been shown to inhibit development of cancers like breast, liver, stomach, lung and colon in rats. Cauliflower also contains anti-inflammatory compounds that help to keep a check on inflammation related diseases. Choline, one of the B vitamins found in good quantity in cauliflower, is vital for cognitive functioning of the brain. Lastly, cauliflower detoxifies the body, and reduces oxidative stress.

Celery: Tropical Celery Tornado

Celery juice is a very hydrating food. It is also alkalizing and balances the body's pH which is an essential component for good health. During ancient times celery was considered to be a medicinal herb useful for treating different health issues.

Celery sticks are bunched together around a tender centre and range in colour from white to dark green. The darker colour is an indication of stronger flavour. It may be consumed raw in salads or cooked. Uncooked celery is mildly bitter with a crisp texture. Its perfect balance of potassium and sodium promotes urine and aids in removal of excess water and uric acid form the body.

Celery is also one of the few foods that is known to bring on severe allergic reactions for people who are allergic to it. It may cause potentially fatal anaphylactic shock. The allergen responsible is not destroyed in cooking. The root of the vegetable, the part put into drinks, contains greater quantities of the allergen compared to the stalk itself.

Tropical Celery Tornado Ingredients:

- ½ cup cubed papaya
- ½ cup cubed pineapple
- ½ cup cubed mango
- 4 stalks of celery

Juice all ingredients and drink immediately to attain maximum nutritional value.

Add-ons

- Kiwi
- Celery leaves

Nutritional Information

Celery stems are a great source of vitamin C, K, B1, B2 and B6. Additionally it is a good supplier of potassium, calcium, folate, iron, magnesium, molybdenum, phosphorus, sodium and loads of essential amino acids. Consuming celery raw also adds plenty of fibre.

Unlike table salt, which is harmful for individuals with high blood pressure, organic sodium in celery is safe even for people with high blood pressure or are otherwise sensitive to salt. Unlike a lot of foods which lose their nutritional value upon cooking, majority of the nutrients in celery maintain their strength.

Health Benefits of Celery

Two special compounds, luteolin and polyacetylenes present in celery in large quantities are beneficial for inflammation related diseases like osteoporosis, arthritis, gout as well as asthma. Luteolin has been shown in studies to be an inhibitor of some enzymes that promote inflammation while polyacetylenes lower levels of prostaglandins, another type of inflammation causing compound. The compound phthalide found in celery aids in relaxing muscles inside blood vessels thus aiding in lowering blood pressure. The excessive levels of coumarines in celery lower the effect of stress causing hormones cortisol in the body. Too much cortisol in the body tightens blood vessels and puts circulatory system under stress. While celery is loaded with potent antioxidants and flavonols that fight cancer, the flavonoids apigenin and luteolin have especially been linked with helping to stop cancer in scientific studies. Consumption of celery juice also helps to detoxify the body, benefit the skin, and provide vital electrolytes when the body is dehydrated.

Cherry: Velvety Cherry Smoothie

This sweet and sour fruit is loaded with antioxidants and polyphenols that help fight disease and aid in improving overall health.

Two main varieties of cherries are available in the market, sweet and sour and not all of them are created equal. Sweet cherries are higher in calories and lower in vitamin C and beta-carotene compared to sour cherries. Regardless, of the type you prefer, the fruit is bursting with goodness.

Cherries are known as a drupe fruit, meaning a fleshy part called the exocarp, surrounds a hard shell or pit and is typically around 2 cm in diameter. The fruit has a very thin, shiny peel that ranges from light red to deep red and purple in colour. Cherries trees have a very short fruiting season in the summer months and grow in most temperate climates.

Velvety Cherry Smoothie Ingredients:

- 1 cup fresh, pitted cherries
- 1 large frozen banana
- 1/2 cup milk
- Honey (optional)

Place the milk and banana into a blender and run for 30 seconds. Add the pitted cherries and blend for one more minute or until the fruit is velvety smooth.

Add-ons

- Cucumber
- Yoghurt

Nutritional Information

Cherries are a high fiber food, delivering 8 per-cent of the daily recommended allowance in just a single 73 gram serving. The same serving also provides 12 grams of carbohydrates, 10 grams of sugar, 1 gram of protein, no cholesterol, sodium or saturated fat and only 50 calories. They also provide significant amounts of vitamin C, A, B6, and K. They are not lacking in minerals either, delivering small amounts of manganese, copper, iron, calcium, zinc, phosphorus and magnesium. Lastly, cherries are a good source of beta-carotene and phytosterols.

Health Benefits of Cherries

Cherries provide some unique medicinal benefits. They contain compounds that have the capacity to relieve pain better than certain commercial drugs like ibuprofen or aspirin. The antioxidant, anthocyanins also responsible for the colour of the fruit, exhibit anti-inflammatory properties which help to cut down on pain associated with arthritis and gout. Additionally the compound behaves like a brain tonic. It helps to avert dementia and Alzheimer and is associated with enhanced insulin production which is of benefit to people with diabetes. Melatonin, another nutrient in cherries acts like an insomnia drug, allowing you to get to sleep faster.

Coriander: Minty Cilantro & Coriander seed Juice

Coriander (seeds) and Cilantro (the green leaves and stems) is a potent herb with a wide range of health benefits. It is also one of the very limited numbers of herbs used for heavy metal detoxification, like mercury, lead, aluminium and cadmium and others.

Coriander seeds as well as cilantro are known as dhania on the Indian Continent. Coriander leaves are employed as herb to add flavour and garnish food, while the seeds fall in the spice category and can be used whole or powdered. The plant belongs to the carrot family with other members being celery, parsley and cumin. It is one of the most ancient spices known to man. The herb is mentioned in the Bible and its seeds were found among ruins dating 5000 B.C.

Minty Cilantro & Coriander Seeds Juice Ingredients:

- 2 large cucumbers
- 1 bunch cilantro
- 1 lemon
- Honey (optional)

Cut the cucumbers into large chunks and remove the ring of the lemon. Thoroughly wash the cilantro. Juice everything in turns. If desired add the honey according to taste at the end.

Add-ons

- Carrots
- apples

Nutritional Information

A fifty gram serving of cilantro leaves deliver 15% of the recommended daily allowance of vitamin C, 113% of vitamin A, and 129% of vitamin K. It also supplies riboflavin, niacin and folic acid. In the minerals department the leaves are a good source of potassium, manganese, calcium, magnesium and iron. The tips of stems and leaves are a rich source of the antioxidants like beta-caretone, and polyphenolic flavonoids like kaempferol, quercetin, egignenin and rhamnetin. These phytochemicals along with the essential oils like boreol, cineol, cymene land others provide the leaves with fungicidal, digestive, antispasmodic, analgesic and carminative properties.

Health Benefits of Cilantro & Coriander Seeds

The latest studies show that coriander is beneficial in treating depression, and anxiety due to its anxiolytic and sedative properties. The linalool oil found in the plant helps to detoxify the liver and enhance appetite. It also has blood thinning properties and medicinal teas made with the seeds can be used in treating indigestion.

Cilantro contain antibiotic compound which when tested in a laboratory proved to be twice as effective as the common drug for killing food-borne bacteria, salmonella. The wide ranging anti-oxidants in cilantro help to reduce the risk of oxidative stress in cells that can lead to cancer. The calcium in cilantro is beneficial for healthy bones while studies with mice show the herb to have anti-diabetic properties and help to control blood sugar. Regular juicing and consumption can stimulate the secretion of insulin and lower bad cholesterol. The elevated levels of beta-carotene in cilantro help to improve eyesight and reduce age related eye problems like cataract.

Just one ounce of cilantro juice one its own or mixed with other juices is sufficient to make noticeable improvements in brain function.

Cranberries: Thick Cranberry Smoothie

Cranberries are an essential component for all-round wellbeing. They are especially rich in the antioxidants, proanthocyanidin and numerous other chemical substances that offer protection against a wide array of ailments.

Cranberries are hard and tend to be very tart hence; eating them out of hand is not suitable for all tastes. Typically they are sold in the dried and sweetened form. Approximately 95% of the cranberry crop is processed and employed in making cranberry juice or sauce. Even the juice is combined with other fruits to cut down on its natural tart flavour.

To ensure that the freshest berries are processed an innovative discovery was made by John Web, a New Jersey grower. Rather than carrying the fruit down the steps of his barn he slid them down to discover that only the firmest and most fresh berries made it all the way down to the last step. The rotting or bruised berries stayed on the steps. This idea was used to develop the bounce board separators that are used even today to separate the good berries from poor quality ones.

Thick Cranberry Smoothie Ingredients:

- 1 frozen banana
- ½ cup fresh cranberries
- ½ cup low fat yoghurt
- 1 tbsp. honey
- ½ cup ice

Cut the banana into pieces and place in the blender with all the other ingredients. Blend all ingredients until velvety smooth.

Add-ons

- apple

Nutritional Information

Not only are cranberries low in calories, making them the ideal health food, but one serving of 100 grams provides 0.39 milligrams of protein, 4.04 milligrams of sugar,0.13 milligrams of fat, 4.6 milligrams of fibre and no cholesterol. They are full of vitamins A, B1, B2, B3, B5, B6, and vitamin C. In the mineral department, cranberries are certainly not lacking in any way with calcium, magnesium, zinc, phosphorus, iron, potassium, manganese, phosphorus, copper, selenium and sodium.

Health Benefits of Cranberries

Cranberries are most widely recognized for their ability to prevent urinary track infects. However, most recent research shows them to be useful in a variety of other ailments. The proanthocyanidins that help prevent UTI also benefit oral health by inhibiting bacteria from binding to teeth and gums and eliminating plaque build-up that leads to gum disease and tooth decay.

The antioxidants in cranberries neutralize free radicals in the body and protect the cells against damage. In turn this prevents the growth of tumors that may lead to cancers of the breast, prostate, colon or lung. The anti-bacterial characteristics of cranberries kill bacteria and stop its growth in the stomach thus proving to be helpful in preventing ulcers. The Phytonutrients and flavonoids in cranberries aid in improving overall stomach health. Lastly, the vitamin C in the fruit helps to enhance immunity against common diseases like fever, cough, and colds.

Cucumber: Quick Hydrating Cucumber Juice

Cucumbers are at times referred to as super-foods due to the wealth of vital nutrients they provide. They are low in calories and contain 96% water, making them the ideal choice for people wishing to lose weight.

The humble cucumber hardly gets any glory, yet it is one of the most widely cultivated vegetables in the world, well technically it is a fruit. It is also among the oldest foods on the planet, associated with the legend of Gilgamesh and listed as one of the foods of ancient Ur.

Cucumbers are the one ingredient you can easily combine in all juicing recipes. Its mild taste goes well with everything without adding any overpowering flavor or aroma of its own. Cucumbers yield plenty of juice making it the ultimate compliment to fruits and vegetables that don't yield a lot of juice. The whole thing can be juiced, seeds, flesh and skin, thus eliminating the trouble of peeling. As a matter of fact the skin and seeds contain more nutrients than the flesh.

Quick Hydrating Cucumber Juice Ingredients:

- 1 large cucumber
- 1 pear
- 1 handful fresh mint

Thoroughly wash all ingredients and cut the cucumber and pear into pieces small enough to fit your juicer with ease. There is no need to remove the peel. Juice the mint first followed by the cucumber and pears.

Add-ons

- Apple
- ginger

Nutritional Information

Cucumber is a rich source of the clotting vitamin, otherwise known as vitamin K with a half a cup serving delivering almost 10 per cent of the requirement of an adult. A half cup of sliced cucumbers also provides significant amounts of vitamins A, C, folate, riboflavin, iron, manganese, magnesium, pantothenic acid, phosphorus and potassium. It contains no saturated fats, cholesterol or sugar and is low in sodium. Furthermore, cucumbers are loaded with Phyto-nutrients carotene ß, xanthin-ß, Lutein.

Health Benefits of Cucumber

Cucumber juice is frequently recommended as a source of silica if improving skin complexion, hair and nail health is the goal; its high water content makes it a good hydrating drink. Silica is also a vital part of healthy connective tissue inclusive of muscles, ligaments, cartilage, tendons and bone. Applied to the skin topically it takes care of a host of skin problems like swelling under the eyes and sunburn. The ascorbic acid and caffeic acid in cucumbers averts water retention.

Cucumbers contain plant lignans, in the digestive tract these bind with bacteria converting them into enterolignans for estrogenic effects. This reduces the risks of estrogen linked cancers like ovary, breast, prostate and uterus. The cucurbitacins in cucumbers block cancer cell development.

Dandelion: Hardy Dandelion Greens Juice

Regardless of the fact that most people hate to see dandelions growing in their yards, this little plant has some very potent health benefits.

Although a weed technically, in the natural health circles it is more commonly referred to as "dandelion greens". Everyone from the Celts to Romans understood the value of this plan and consumed it as food. Dandelions were a standard plant cultivated in monasteries for its medicinal value, and even Arab doctors recommended it for various ailments. Today it is commonly used throughout Europe as a diuretic and a number of other ailments. Typically all of the leaves emerging from below the flower can be juice or eaten in other ways.

Hardy Dandelion Greens Juice Ingredients:

- 1 large handful dandelion leaves
- 1 celery stick
- ½ lemon
- 2 apples

Wash all ingredients and chop into pieces small enough to fit your juicer. Juice all the ingredients starting with dandelion leaves and serve over ice.

Add-ons

- Pear
- Cucumber

Nutritional Information

The common dandelion plant contains more nutrients than most vegetables available in the grocery store. Two cups have only 45 calories but provide 203% of the daily requirement of vitamin A, 58% vitamin C, 17% iron and 20% calcium. Additionally it is an outstanding source of vitamins K, E, B6, thiamin, manganese, potassium and riboflavin. It is also a good source of folate, copper, magnesium and phosphorus. The phytochemical taraxacin in dandelion is understood to be the source of dandelion's tonic like effects on the digestion. Its abundant supply of antioxidants and other micronutrients provide it with expectorant, antiseptic, and germicidal effects.

Health Benefits of Dandelions

Dandelions are loaded with usable calcium which is essential for bone strength and growth. The antioxidants like vitamin C and Luteolin offer protection against age-related bone damage such as decreased bone density. These same nutrients keep the liver functioning at optimal levels while other compounds found in dandelions protect it against hemorrhaging. Dandelions regulate the flow of bile and incite the liver to enhance digestion.

Diabetes is a major health issue in the world today. Dandelion juice stimulates the production of insulin and helps in maintaining blood sugar levels in the normal range. Being diuretic in nature, dandelions also help to remove toxic substances from the body by increasing urination. The disinfectant characteristics of the plant help to eliminate microbial development in the urinary system. Sap from dandelion is beneficial in treating skin diseases resulting from fungal and microbial infections.

Fennel: Fennel Juice Fusion

It is said that when it comes to juicing you can't go wrong with fennel. Its anti-fungal and bacterial characteristics combined with sweet taste make it a good juice to have on a regular basis.

Fennel has been used as a medicinal plant since the Greek times, in fact it was their belief that the plant had the ability to pass knowledge from gods to man. It was traditionally used in Europe for digestive disorders.

Funnel juice blends well with a wide range of ingredients like pears, apples, carrots and cucumber. Its aniseed like flavor adds a very distinctive flavor to the juice. In juicing, the root bulb of the plant is used most of the time however its stems and fronds can also be used. If you find the aroma and flavor to be a bit over powering, then start with just half a bulb added to other fruits or vegetables to take advantage of all its benefits.

Funnel Juice Fusion Ingredients:

- 2 medium sized green apples (or equivalent)
- 2 sticks celery with leaves
- 1 bulb funnel, can include stems

Chop all ingredients to a size that will easily fit your juicer. Run them through the juicer and enjoy the juice as soon after juicing as possible over ice.

Add-ons

- Lemon
- kale

Funnel Nutritional Information

This seemingly average herb is loaded with some very potent nutrients. It is an exceptional source of vitamin C, folate, manganese, and potassium. Additionally it is a good source of iron, niacin, calcium and magnesium. It also contains phytoestrogens making it useful in the relief of menopause symptoms and the oil anethole which provides anti-inflammatory benefits.

Health Benefits of Fennel

Funnel contains aspartic acid which gives it carminative properties. It is commonly used as an anti-flatulent and is safe enough even for infants. In fact it is used to treat colic babies. The iron and histidine, an amino acid, help in the formation of blood components. Chewing on fennel seeds after a meal stimulates the secretion of digestive juices that aid digestion and eliminate bad breath. Powdered fennel seeds act as a laxative. The potassium in fennel is a good vasodilator, meaning it relaxes the blood vessels and aids in reducing blood pressure. Additionally potassium is an electrolyte which facilitates electrical conduction in the body.

The cineole and anetol present in fennel behave like expectorants aiding in respiratory disorders like bronchitis and congestion. Fennel helps to break apart phlegm making breathing easier. Fennel is also a diuretic which aids in removal of toxins from the body.

Fig: Fig Almond Smoothie

Sweet nutty flavour and delicate in aroma, figs are loaded with calcium, fibre and antioxidants. A fig smoothie makes for the perfect breakfast drink or a replenishing mid-day snack.

Fig trees are among the oldest trees on the planet. They feature prominently in the Bible and were held in such high esteem by the Greeks that at one point in time laws were established to prevent their export. The fig fruit has a soft somewhat chewy texture with edible seeds scattered throughout the fruit. While fresh figs are delicate and have a short shelf life, they can easily be dried for long time preservation.

Fig Almond Smoothie Ingredients:

- 3 fresh figs (dried can also be used)
- 1 cup coconut milk
- 10 almonds
- 1 tsp. honey (optional)
- ½ cup ice

Wash and cut the figs into halves. Add all ingredients into a blender and blend for 40-50 seconds, or until a desired smoothness is reached. Enjoy the energizing drink.

Add-ons

- Dates
- Pecans
- Cinnamon

Nutritional Information

Fresh figs are approximately 80% water and a hundred gram serving provides roughly 74 calories. The same serving also delivers almost no fat, no cholesterol, close to twenty grams of carbohydrates, sixteen grams of sugar and three grams of dietary fiber. It also houses many important vitamins including vitamins A, B6, C, E, K, thiamin, riboflavin niacin and folates. In the mineral department, it is a rich source of potassium, calcium, magnesium, and phosphorus with trace amounts of iron, sodium and zinc.

Health Benefits of Figs

Studies indicate that consumption of figs increases the body's antioxidant ability for up to four hours after consumption. The darker coloured varieties have greater antioxidant capabilities with a large number of the phytonutrients housed in the skin of the ripe fruit. These antioxidants prevent oxidation of the lipoproteins in the blood and reduce overall oxidative stress of the body. Just three medium sized figs deliver five grams of fibre which helps to prevent constipation and overall digestive health. Additionally figs contain prebiotics that are beneficial for the friendly bacteria in the intestine, further aiding digestive system. The flavonoid quercetin is linked with averting lung and colon cancer. Luteolin, another flavonoid in figs has anti-inflammatory properties and is very good at impeding growth of tumours. Topical application of luteolin has been shown to prevent and treat skin cancer. Figs contain a lot of potassium, which acts to relax blood vessels and helps to control blood pressure.

Garlic: Garlic Veggie Juice

Not many people drink vegetable juices for their taste, but there is no denying of the benefits offered by the elixir made with a variety of beautifully blended vegetables spiked with garlic. In fact, according to folk medicine garlic was believed to have been the cure for everything from the Plague to the common cold.

The underground bulb of the garlic plant is the most commonly used portion of the plant. It is an essential component of most dishes prepared in Asia, Middle East, North Africa, Southern Europe and parts of South America. The bulb is divided into many sections known as cloves, which may be consumed raw, used in cooking or as medicine. Other parts of the plant like the leaves and flowers may also be consumed. They have a milder flavor than the bulbs.

The pungent, spicy taste of the bulbs softens and sweetens as cooked. Many people find raw garlic to be a bit aggressive for their tastes. However, combined with some mild and sweet tasting green vegetables in juices, its sting can be minimized and the taste pleasing.

Garlic Veggie Juice Ingredients:

- 2 cloves garlic
- ½ an avocado
- 1 medium cucumber
- 1 small green apple
- few mint leaves

Add-ons

- carrot
- celery

Nutritional Information

Garlic is a good source of calcium, selenium, vitamin B1 and phosphorus and a very good source of vitamin C, B6, copper and manganese. It is very low in calories, saturated fat, sodium and cholesterol. It also contains some thiamin, riboflavin pantothenic acid, iron, magnesium, potassium, zinc and omega-3 and 6 fatty acids.

Allicin is one of garlic's most valuable sulfur compounds. It works best for your health if you chop or crush fresh garlic clove and allow it to sit for a few minutes at room temperature, before cooking it or using it in a juice. If the garlic clove is cooked whole or even a mild acid like lemon juice is added to it, it will lose some of its anti-cancer properties.

Health Benefits of Garlic

According to an old folk remedy, eating a clove of garlic dipped in honey at the first sign of a cold will ward off colds and flu. Modern medical studies indicate that garlic boosts the immune system and fights chest infections, congestion and coughs. US and European studies have shown that garlic reduces the levels of bad cholesterol in the blood and aids babies in the womb to gain weight. Garlic is also known to be a potent antioxidant that protects the body against free radical damage as well as the bacterium Helicobacter pylori, a leading stomach ulcer causing bacteria. One San Francisco area study found that garlic reduced risks of pancreatic cancer while a study in France linked greater consumption of garlic with lower risks of breast cancer.

Ginger: Spunky Ginger Smoothie

Ginger is a popular herb with important culinary and medicinal value. It holds a special place in Chinese and Indian medicines due to its unique phytochemicals with health enhancing properties.

An underground rhizome, ginger flesh can be found in red, white or yellow color depending on the variety. Even though ginger is commonly available in the dried form in supermarkets, fresh ginger is superior in flavor and it contains greater amounts of gingerol, an active protease responsible for ginger's anti-inflammatory quality. It can also be purchased in candied, pickled and crystallized forms. Ginger works equally well in fruit and green smoothies, adding a spicy, warming flavor. It also works well when used in combination with other spices like nutmeg and cinnamon.

Spunky Ginger Smoothie Ingredients:

- 4 tsp fresh grated ginger root
- 1 large red delicious apple
- 1 small cucumber
- 1 cups dandelion greens
- 8 ounces almond milk

Add the almond milk, ginger and apple into a blender and turn it on for about 20 seconds. Add all the greens and continue blending another 30-40 seconds. Enjoy over ice.

Add-ons

- Papaya
- Celery

Nutritional Information

One quarter cup of ginger provides 0.2 grams of fat, 0.4 grams of protein, 0.5 grams of fibre, 4.3 grams of carbohydrates and 19 calories. It also delivers 2% of the daily recommended amounts of vitamin B6, and C while supplying limited amounts of riboflavin, niacin, folate, thiamine and vitamin E. Ginger in not lacking in the minerals department either. It is a rich source of potassium, magnesium, manganese and copper, in addition to supplying small amounts of calcium, iron, zinc and phosphorus. Ginger is especially valued for the antioxidants known as gingerals and is also a source of omega-3 and 6 fatty acids.

Health Benefits of Ginger

Ginger offers a number of health benefits, but is especially recognized for gingerals which deter the formation of inflammation causing compounds in the body. Clinical studies show that ¾ of the arthritis and 100% of the patients suffering from muscular pain obtained relief by taking only ¼ inch slice of ginger on a regular basis. Adding ginger to drinks offers anticoagulant benefits. It also reduces the stickiness of blood platelets which provides protection against the risk of atherosclerosis. National Library of Medicine, a department of the National Institute of Health, U.S.A, reports that ginger is utilized to treat appetite loss, post-surgery nausea and vomiting, flatulence, colic, morning sickness and upset stomach throughout the world.

Grape: Green Grape Smoothie

Grapes blend pleasantly with most other fruits and add an appetizing flavour to green smoothies also. Consumption of grapes offers numerous health benefits with studies associating them to prevention of serious diseases like cardiovascular disorders, cancer and elevated blood pressure.

Grapes are available in numerous colours from white to red, black green golden and purple. They are classified as a type of a berry with leather like cover and a moist flesh inside. Fresh grapes are approximately eighty per-cent water and low in calories, making them a good diet snack, while raisins (dried grapes) only have about fifteen per-cent water. This means the nutrients are much more densely packed in raisins which is why one cup has close to eight times more calories. Grapes are however high in sugars, hence people with diabetes need to proceed with caution, but this very fact makes them a good moderate addition to green smoothies.

Green Grape Smoothie Ingredients:

- 2 cups green grapes (may substitute other varieties)
- 1 whole banana
- 1 small handful of fresh Italian parsley
- 2 cups fresh baby spinach (or other leafy green)
- 1/2 cup water if needed

Add-ons

- Pear
- Cucumber

Nutritional Information

A one cup serving, roughly 32 – 35 grapes, provide approximately 100 calories in addition to protein, two per-cent of the daily recommended amount of fibre, two per-cent of the recommend amount of vitamin C, A, iron and calcium. They contain no sodium or saturated fats. They also supply eight per-cent of the daily recommended amount of potassium and carbohydrates.

The poly-phenolic pigments in grapes provide the colour. Dark coloured grapes like red or purple are richer in anti-oxidants anthocyanins while the lighter coloured on like white-green contain more tannins particularly catechin. Other antioxidants found in the berry include resveratrol, lutein and zeaxanthin. It is interesting to note that most of the antioxidants are found in the seeds and skin of the fruit. They also contain some important flavonoids like myricetin and quercetin.

Health Benefits of Grapes

The antioxidant resveratrol fond mostly in the skin of grapes, particularly in the red variety, is linked with slowing down of the aging process of the brain, heart, and other vital organs. At the cellular level it eliminates free radicals and protects healthy DNA. Research has also found that resveratrol may be beneficial for treating Alzheimer's disease, providing relief from mood swings linked with menopause, and aiding in blood glucose control.

Being 60 to 70 percent water, grapes are a good hydrating food, and yield a mildly laxative influence on metabolism. The fiber in the fruit further aids in regulating bowel movements and eradicating constipation. The polyphenols are known to slow and even avert cancers of lung esophagus, mouth, prostate, pancreas and colon. The flavonoid quercetin in grapes are naturally anti-inflammatory and help in cutting down the risks of atherosclerosis and harm created by LDL cholesterol, additionally it too may offer anti-cancer benefits.

Grapefruit: Sweet & Sour Grapefruit Juice

Grapefruit is claimed to be a fruit of "paradise" due to the unique health-enhancing and disease fighting properties it possesses. A versatile gem, its peels are used as garnish for dishes while the fruit itself may be juiced or enjoyed whole.

Botanists believe that the grapefruit was created by crossing a Pummelo (the largest citrus fruit) with a sweet orange. It is available in a variety of colours like pink, yellow, ruby and white. The colouration is the result of fruit pigmentation representing the degree of ripeness. Looking at grapefruits growing on trees, one sees a strong resemblance between the way clusters of grapefruits grow and grape clusters, hence the name. The fruit typically ranges from four to six inches in diameter and is a rich source of phytonutrients.

Sweet & Sour Grapefruit Juice Ingredients:

- 1 organic grapefruit
- 1 teaspoon honey

Cut the grapefruit in half and juice manually in a citrus juicer. Blend in the honey and enjoy over ice.

Add-ons

- Carrots
- Dates

Nutritional Information

One half of an approximately four inch diameter grapefruit contains 41 calories. It delivers only one calorie from fat, no cholesterol or sodium. This serving also delivers 5.6 grams of dietary fibre, 4.6 grams of carbohydrates, and almost nine grams of sugar. The same serving provides nearly 60% of the daily requirements of vitamin C, and almost 6.5% of vitamin A. Additionally it supplies fair amounts of vitamin B1, B2, B6, biotin, choline and folate as well as pantothenic acid along with trace amounts of vitamin E. Grapefruits are a good source of potassium and copper while fair sources of magnesium, phosphorus, manganese, and calcium. They also house a number of phytochemicals like lycopene and liminoids.

Grapefruits have a bad reputation when it comes to interacting with certain medications. In fact research indicates that there are 85 drugs with which grapefruit reacts negatively. The chemicals called furanocoumarins in grapefruit block an enzyme in the intestine which metabolises lots of medicines. The net result is that more of these medications get absorbed into the body, making them stronger and leading to undesirable side effects. If you are on any medication, it is best to check with your doctor to ensure that it does not interact with grapefruit.

Health Benefits of Grapefruits

Being an exceptional source of vitamin C, grapefruit helps to support a strong immune system. It also averts the damage caused by free radicals by eliminating them thus preventing the inflammatory surge they cause. Inflammation is the cause of serious diseases like osteoarthritis, asthma, and rheumatoid arthritis. Free radicals left in the body can oxidize cholesterol and result in plaque build-up in the arteries, which is the forerunner of heart attacks and stroke. The lycopene in grapefruit is linked with anti-tumor properties. Consumption of foods rich in lycopene can reduce the risk of prostate cancer according to latest research. The limonoids in the fruit also prevent tumour formation by promoting the production of a detoxifying enzyme that makes toxic substances in the body more water soluble and hence easier to remove. The pectin in grapefruit lowers cholesterol as well as slowing the process of atherosclerosis.

Green Beans: Green Bean Juice

Frequently called "poor man's meat", this fat-free, nutrient rich food should really be called "healthy man's meat". The tiny beans hidden inside an edible pod provide a wealth of health benefits.

Green beans are also referred to as string beans due to the string running lengthwise along the pod seam (which has long since been eliminated by breeding methods), hence its newer name snap beans. They are so called because the newer varieties are picked at a more immature stage and can actually be snapped in two with a simple finger twist action. At times they are also called "haricot vert" which is French for "green beans".

Regardless of the name you call them by, the fact remains that they are easily juiced and provide a mildly sweet flavor to almost any combination of juices. They are relatively inexpensive and easily available throughout the year in most parts of the world.

Green Bean Juice Ingredients:

- 2 cups chopped green beans
- 1 cup chopped spinach
- 1 cucumber
- 1 pear
- 1 tsp lemon juice

Wash all the ingredients thoroughly and chop into appropriate size to fit the juicer with ease. Juice and enjoy chilled with ice.

Add-ons

- Celery
- Kale
- apple

Nutritional Information

Green beans are an exceptional source of a large number of vitamins and minerals. They also provide a number of very important carotenoids like lutein, beta-carotene and zeaxanthin that offer numerous health benefits. A one cup serving of raw green beans contains only 44 calories and provides approximately 22% vitamin K, 18% manganese, 16% vitamin C, 16% fiber (when fiber is not extracted), 10% folate, 9% vitamin B2, 8% copper, 7.5% vitamin B1, 6% chromium, 5% magnesium, potassium, phosphorus, choline, vitamin A , B3 and calcium. Furthermore it supplies 4.5% iron and protein and close to 4% of the daily recommended dose of vitamin E and B6.

Health Benefits of Green Beans

When looking at green beans you would never guess that they contain the same pigments which give some vegetables their yellow, orange and red colors. While the main function of these compounds is to work as antioxidants, they carry out other jobs as well. The beta-carotene is converted into a form of vitamin A necessary for normal night vision, while lutein and zeaxanthin protect the eyes against high intensity light. The calcium you consume is only good for the bones if it is absorbed by the body. Vitamin K makes proteins necessary for the absorption of calcium. Additionally it regulates bone metabolism to maintain bone density. The vitamin C offers protection to healthy cells against damage from free radicals. Vitamin C is also used by the body to produce collagen which is needed for young looking skin, healthy tendons, connective tissue, bone and organs. The manganese in green beans relieves symptoms of osteoporosis, and PMS, while helping the body to absorb other vital nutrients.

Jerusalum Artichoke: Cleansing Jerusalem artichoke

The Jerusalem artichoke can never achieve star status in juicing recipes rather due to its bland taste; it makes an exceptional additive so you can take full advantage of its valuable nutrients.

Also going by the name of earth apple, Sunroot, Sunchoke and Topinambour, the Jerusalem artichoke shares no other connections with the holy city besides the name. Furthermore, it is not even a true artichoke! It was originally cultivated by the American Indians and is in reality a type of sunflower. The name is obtained from the Italian word girasole meaning sunflower.

Cleansing Jerusalem artichoke Juice

- 1 cup chopped Jerusalem artichokes
- 1 small cucumber
- 1 apple
- 2 carrots

Add-ons

- Kale leaves
- ginger

Nutritional Information

Jerusalem artichoke supplies the greatest amounts of iron among the typically eaten roots and tubers. A one hundred gram serving of the fresh vegetable fulfils about 42% of the daily iron needs. It is also a very good source of potassium and magnesium, two important electrolytes, in addition to phosphorous. The tuber also contains small quantities of the anti-oxidant vitamins such as vitamin C, A and E. Furthermore, it contains small amounts of the group of B-complex vitamins like folates, riboflavin, pantothenic acid, pyridoxine and thiamin.

The Jerusalem artichoke makes a good supplement to any diet plan since one gram contributes only 73 calories, a significant 1.6 grams of fibre, only 0.01 grams of fat and two grams of protein.

Health Benefits of Jerusalem artichoke

Artichokes offer many advantages. They contain a carbohydrate called inulin, which impersonates insulin and breaks down into fructose in the colon. This does not affect blood sugar levels like carbohydrates that break down into glucose. This makes the vegetable diabetic friendly. Inulin is also considered a prebiotic as it is not easily digested and is food for the friendly bacteria residing in the large intestine. Additionally, inulin has been known to provide relief from constipation by adding bulk to the digestive tract. Finally, it aides calcium absorption, cuts down on levels of triglycerides and LDL cholesterol, as well as obstruct a variety of cancers.

Jicama: Nutty Jicama Juice

This, not so common an ingredient in the U.S, is a delicious option for juicing with a flavor that is a cross between an apple and a potato. Rich in nutrients, its juice compliments a range of flavors.

Jicama, a root vegetable that is traditionally a common addition to salsas and salads, is now fast becoming a favored ingredient in smoothies and juices due to the variety of key nutrients it offers. While it looks somewhat like a turnip, in reality it is a member of the legume family. Most of the vital nutrients are near the skin, so it is advisable to remove only a very thin layer of the skin before juicing. Jicama juice is mild in flavor but thick and creamy in appearance.

Nutty Jicama Juice Ingredients

- 1 cup strawberries
- 1 small Jicama (without the brown skin)
- 1 small cucumber
- 1 Chinese pear
- 2 sprigs mint, plus some leaves for garnish

Add-ons

- Honey
- Carrots

Nutritional Information

A single cup of jicama houses 0.78 milligrams of iron. This satisfies nearly 4% of the daily iron requirements for women. It additionally supplies magnesium, potassium and manganese. It also contains additional minerals like zinc, calcium and selenium in minor quantities. The same quantity also delivers 35% of vitamin C needed by women daily, along with small quantities of folate, and vitamins A and E.

Jicama is also a good source of phytonutrients, the plant-based compounds with strong antioxidant abilities. This includes inhibiting free radicals from damaging DNA and cell tissue as well as offering other health benefits. Jicama is also a good source of soluble fiber, with a 100 gram serving fulfilling 13% of the daily needs.

Health Benefits of Jicama

The elevated amounts of vitamin C in jicama offer potent anti-inflammatory properties, which help to eliminate asthma symptoms like wheezing, particularly in children. Additionally it helps to keep colds and flu at bay. Being a good source of fiber, jicama helps to maintain low cholesterol and stable sugar levels. Raw jicama is a low calorie food containing only 35 calories in a 100 gram serving; this makes it good for people wishing to lose weight.

The amino acid homocysteine is one of the factors for heart disease and linked with renal disease. Jicama is known to cut down on the levels of this amino acid and in turn reduce the risks of heart and renal disease.

Kale: Bone Forming Kale Smoothie

Kale has been treasured for its highly nutritious properties since the ancient times of Greeks and Romans. It has gained greater popularity in the last few years as a green juice and smoothie ingredient and is a favored drink of many health conscious celebrities.

Kale belongs to the cabbage family and comes in two varieties. One has smooth leaves and the other more common variety comes with leaves that are wrinkled and is known as curly kale. Kale leaves do not form heads instead they develop on top of individual stems. They are usually dark green colored but at times also have blue or purple ting to them.

Kale along with other cruciferous vegetables is thought to be goiter causing if taken in excessive amounts. However, used in moderation with a well-balanced diet, it offers more benefits than harm.

Bone Forming Kale Smoothie Ingredients:

- 1 avocado
- A generous handful of kale
- 1 cup pineapple pieces
- 1 small cucumber
- 250ml coconut water

Wash the kale thoroughly, peel and dice the cucumber, pineapple and avocado. Place all the fruit and vegetables in a blender, top off with the coconut water and blend to smoothness.

Add-ons

- Spanish onion

Nutritional Information

One cup of kale contains only 36 calories and delivers a whopping 5 grams of fiber along with many vital vitamins and antioxidants. Research shows that the vegetable contains 45 flavonoids offering numerous antioxidant and anti-inflammatory benefits.

Furthermore, the USDA National Nutrient data base reports that only 100 grams of kale supplies more than 650% of the daily requirement of vitamin K, more than 500% of vitamin A, 200% vitamin C, in addition to small amounts of folates, niacin, pantothenic acid, pyridoxine, riboflavin, and thiamin. It also delivers a range of minerals like copper, manganese, iron, calcium, phosphorus and magnesium. Trace amounts of zinc, and selenium are also present.

Health Benefits of Kale

New research shows the many benefits of kale. The broad spectrum of antioxidants present and very high amounts of vitamin K along with a kind of vitamin E have been shown to reduce cholesterol and perhaps also play a role in lowering the risks of some cancers. The indole-3-carbinol in kale has a role in the way estrogen is metabolized in the body which offers natural protection against breast cancer and other estrogen-dominant diseases like endometriosis or fibroids.

The elevated amounts of vitamin C increases metabolism to help with weight loss and strengthens the immune system by fighting viruses and bacteria. Kale contains more iron than beef, which is good news for vegans as iron aids in supplying more oxygen to the blood and fighting anemia. A healthy balance of omega-3 and 6 fatty acids in kale helps to fight autoimmune diseases like arthritis and asthma while the folic acid and vitamin B6 offer cardiovascular benefits to fight heart disease.

Kiwi: Wholesome Kiwi Smoothie

Kiwifruit has been used by the ancient Chinese as a health tonic since ancient times. The emerald colored fruit contains a large variety of health promoting phytonutrients.

A native of China, the kiwifruit was carried to New Zealand by missionaries at the start of the twentieth century. Originally known as Yang Tao, it was renamed Chinese Gooseberries in 1960. The goose berries were first brought to public notice in United States after being served in a restaurant in 1961.

The oval-shaped fruit features a brown skin with fuzzy hairs. Inside is the semitransparent, emerald green flesh housing white veins lying in concentric arrangement and tiny black seeds. Somewhat creamy in consistency, the fruit tastes like a cross between strawberries and bananas.

Wholesome Kiwi Smoothie Ingredients:

- 1 cup diced kiwifruit
- 3 tablespoons porridge oats
- 1 medium sized banana
- 6 ice cubes
- 200 ml organic milk
- 200 g organic yoghurt
- Honey to taste

Place all ingredients, minus the honey, in a blender and whiz until smooth and creamy (approximately thirty seconds). Pour into glasses, add the honey and enjoy.

Add-ons

- Cinnamon
- Ginger

Nutritional Information

Kiwi fruit is a good source of fiber, with one cup satisfying a little over 20% of the daily fiber needs and no saturated fat or cholesterol. The same serving also delivers more than 270% of the daily requirements of vitamin C, nearly 90% requirements of the vitamin K requirements, 13% vitamin E, 11% foliate, in addition to small amounts of thiamine, riboflavin, niacin, vitamin A and pantothenic acid. It is also a good supplier of copper, potassium, manganese, magnesium, phosphorus and calcium. Lastly, it contains vital carotenoids like lutein, zeaxanthin and beta-carotene.

Health Benefits of Kiwi

Studies have found that it is conceivable for kiwifruit to house properties of a natural blood thinner. According to one finding regular consumption of the fruit reduced triglyceride levels and platelet accumulation in the way aspirin therapy does. This has the potential to cut down on risks involving blood clot. Another published study has found kiwifruit to meaningfully improve insomnia in adults.

The high content of vitamin C in kiwifruit is a vital antioxidant that helps to stop the skin from being harmed by the sun, smoke and pollution, thus preventing premature aging and maintaining healthy skin texture. The generous amounts of potassium and fiber in kiwifruit help to support heart health and possibly reduce blood pressure by negating the effects of sodium. Especially noteworthy is the fact that there is a 20% less chance of dying from any cause if the daily 4700 milligram of potassium intake is met.

Lemon: Sweet & Sour Lemon Smoothie

Lemons are one of the few natural products capable of serving not only culinary or aromatherapy advantages, but medicinal, health and disinfecting purposes as well. Hardly any other natural product serves such a wide variety of purposes.

Belonging to the same family as the orange, grapefruit and tangerine, lemon is valued not only for its juice but the rind as well. While the origins of the lemon lie in the foothills of Himalayas, it is now cultivated around the globe. Its tart juice not only flavors numerous dishes, and provides many important nutrients as well. Various parts of the fruit are also employed in homes to disinfect, remove stains and to dissuade flies, mosquitoes and other pests.

Lemons contain powerful antioxidants known as bioflavonoids. It is believed that these compounds are responsible for the health properties lemons have to offer.

Sweet & Sour Lemon Smoothie Ingredients:

- 1 peeled & seeded lemon
- 1 small apple
- 1 small banana
- 1/4 cup yogurt
- 2 teaspoons honey
- 6 ice cubes

Blend all ingredients except the ice cubes until smooth. Add the ice and blend for another 10 seconds, pour into a glass and enjoy.

Add-ons

- Ginger

* Pear

Nutritional Information

Other than the lack of fat, low sodium, plenty of fiber and nominal calories in a lemon, it also is highly admired for its nutrients and antioxidant properties. Additionally it is now being recognized that other biologically active compounds present in lemon help to cut down on cancer risks, as well as a number of chronic modern ailments.

Lemon is a good source of crucial vitamins which the body must acquire from external sources like pantothenic acid, pyridoxine and folates. In addition to being a plentiful supplier of minerals such as iron, calcium, and potassium, it is also an exceptional source of vitamin C.

Health Benefits of Lemon

Lemons have been used for generations to cure a large number of disorders including throat infections, fever, respiratory problems, internal bleeding, burns and cholera. According to an American Urological Association study, lemon juice prevents formation of kidney stones by producing urinary citrate which does not allow the crystals (stones) to form. The soluble fiber pectin, found in lemons is associated with keeping blood sugar levels stable and fiber in general gives the feeling of being full longer, thus aiding in weight loss.

A "Journal of Food Composition and Analysis" review published in 2006 states that lemons contain large amount of flavanones, phytochemicals that are believed to put a stop to stroke, asthma, cancer, heart disease as well as neurological issues by blocking DNA and cell destroying ability of free radicals. The flavanone, hesperidin helps to maintain strong bones and reduce blood lipid levels and the flavanone, eriocitrin shields the liver against oxidative destruction.

Lettuce: Recharging Lettuce Juice

Lettuce has been known since ancient times for its purifying and refreshing benefits. In modern times, lettuce has become a favored ingredient in green juices.

Lettuce obtains its scientific name from the milky "latex" liquid that seeps out of the stems after being cut. This milky fluid, called 'lectucarium' gives lettuce the mildly bitter taste as well as providing it with medicinal value. The compound delivers sedative like effect of opium, without any of the dangerous consequences. Both the leaf and stem are safe for consumption.

There are numerous varieties and sub-varieties of lettuce available, with the iceberg, butterhead and romaine being the most common. Each variety has its own distinct flavor, texture and keeping qualities. Romaine lettuce offers the most nutritional value while iceberg lettuce contains the minimum amounts.

Recharging Lettuce Juice Ingredients:

- ½ head romaine lettuce
- 2 sticks of celery
- 1 pear
- 1 lemon

Thoroughly wash the ingredients and cut so they fit the juicer easily. Juice all ingredients except lemon; pour in a glass and finally hand squeeze the lemon last. Drink immediately for maximum benefits.

Add-ons

- Apple
- Ginger

Nutritional Information

When thinking of lettuce, the general rule is that the darker green the color, the more nutrient rich it is and the stronger the flavor. Lettuce is 90 to 95 per cent water so it is low in calories, thus making it a good hydrating drink, not to mention the vitamins, minerals and anti-oxidants it is packed with.

A little less than 100 grams of raw lettuce supplies more than 100% of the daily recommended allowance of vitamin K, 45% of vitamin A, nearly 32% of folates, roughly 12% molybdenum, more than 7% manganese, in addition to small amounts of potassium, biotin, copper, iron, phosphorus, chromium, magnesium, calcium, omega-3 fats, vitamins B1, B2, B6, & C, .

Health Benefits of Lettuce

Among the many benefits lettuce provides include its anti-anemic properties. These are due to the excessive amounts of chlorophyll and iron used in the production of red blood cells. The anti-oxidants in the vegetable aide in removing free radicals responsible for damaging healthy cells thereby preventing premature aging and many chronic diseases. It is believed that the high amounts of vitamin K offers protection to bone health, as it is used in production of a bone protein that strengthens bone tissue. Lettuce contains a number of compounds that help to relieve irritating cough in addition to symptoms of bronchitis and asthma.

Mango: Exotic Mango-Fig Smoothie

Supplying a wide array of nutrients coupled with moderate amount of calories makes mangoes not only a healthy food but one that tastes delicious also. Each serving of the tropical fruit is free of sodium, cholesterol and fat, earning them a position in the super fruit category.

Frequently referred to as the "king of fruits" and named one of the most widely consumed fruits in Asia, the mango plants are thought to have originated in the sub-Himalayan plains. The mango fruit is available in numerous shapes, colours and sizes depending on the variety. The unripe green mangoes are pickled, used in chutneys or converted into side dishes, while the ripe fruit can be enjoyed out of hand.

Mangoes have a sweet-juicy flavor with tart under tones. The texture is similar to that of peaches with the best quality fruit containing minimal to no fibers. The size of the fruit varies from two to nine inches with some varieties shaped like a kidney while others are more oval. The center of the fruit contains a single large pit.

Exotic Mango-Fig Smoothie Ingredients:

- 1 cup diced mango pieces.
- 1 cup chopped figs
- ½ cup milk
- 3-4 ice cubes

Place mango, figs and yogurt in a blender. Blend on high speed for 30 seconds. Add in the ice cubes and blend to desired consistency. If the fruit is frozen beforehand, the ice cubes may be omitted. Pour smoothie into glasses and serve.

Add-ons

- Stalk of celery
- Figs

Nutritional Information

One cup of peeled mangoes (225 grams) deliver significant amounts of some important nutrients. They supply 75% of the daily allowance of vitamin C, 25% of the daily vitamin A requirement, 11% of vitamin B6, 9% copper and probiotic fibre, 7% potassium, and 4% magnesium. Additionally it contains smaller amounts of vitamins B2, B1, E, K, niacin, folate, pantothenic acid, phosphorus, calcium, zinc, sodium, iron, selenium, manganese, and magnesium. Mangos also contain many important antioxidants including quercetin, isoquercitrin, lutein, gallic acid, cryptoxanthin, and anacardic acid.

Health Benefits of Mangoes

The pro-biotic fibre and certain enzymes found in mangoes aid digestion. The enzymes break down proteins while the fibrous content helps to clear the digestive tract. The pectin in mangoes is associated with lowering cholesterol levels as well as reducing the risks of prostate cancer. Additionally the host of antioxidants found in mangoes work to protect against leukemia, breast, colon cancers. The fibre content of the fruit combined with the potassium in the fruit help to avert heart disease.

Mint: Minty Mango Smoothie

Medicinal properties of mint have been used in traditional medicine to treat everything from stomach pain and indigestion to whitening teeth and freshening breath. In modern times fresh mint makes the perfect condiment for great tasting, healthy drinks.

While there are around 25 species of mint, peppermint and spearmint are the most common. Typically mints have cool sweet flavor. Peppermint has a strong aroma, and greenish-purple leaves with sharp zig-zag toothed edges, and is the mint that is most commonly employed in commercial use. Spearmint with its grayish green colored leaves that have more rounded, lace-like edges, is most commonly employed for culinary purposes.

All mints contain abundant quantities of volatile oil packed in viscous packets located in the stems and leaves. These oils are utilized as flavoring in food items, perfumery and medicines.

Minty Mango Smoothie Ingredients:

- 1 cup of mango cubes
- 1 medium ripe banana
- 1 cup almond milk
- 10 fresh mint leaves
- 4 – 6 ice cubes
- 1 teaspoon honey

Add-ons

- Yoghurt
- blueberries

Nutritional Information

Like most herbs, mint is low in calories housing only 48 calories in a 100 gram serving. While most of these calories come from carbohydrates, there is also a tiny amount of protein found in mint. It is also low in sodium, saturated fat and cholesterol. Mint is a good source of fiber, containing 2 grams in the said serving. Additionally it is a rich source of carotenes, a nutrient that affords plants their colors and is a forerunner of vitamin A in humans.

Mint is a very good source of vitamin C, vitamin A, along with calcium, iron, folate, and manganese. Furthermore more it contains fair amounts of zinc, niacin, phosphorus, copper, riboflavin and potassium.

Health Benefits of Mint

The benefits of mint kick into operation even before we begin its consumption. The aroma of the leaves triggers salivary glands in the mouth to release digestive enzymes that aid digestion. Controlled studies have shown mint oil to alleviate indigestion, dyspepsia and colonic muscle spasms. The rosmarinic acid in mint gives rise to a number of actions that benefit asthma by keeping airways open for easier breathing. Mint oil is also known to prevent the growth of various bacteria and fungus.

A more recent interest in mint extends to it potential as an anti-cancer agent. The significant amount of the phytonutrient monoerpene present in mint oil has demonstrated its ability to stop mammary, pancreatic and liver tumors in animals. It has also demonstrated protection against skin, colon and lung cancer formation.

Onion: Minty Sweet Onion Juice

Onions have been used as food and medicine around the world for nearly five thousand years. In the middle ages they were used to cure everything from headaches to snake bites and hair loss. Current research shows they can provide relief from a variety of ailments.

The underground onion bulb belonging to the Allium family can be grouped into two main classes; scallions or green onions are not fully ripe and the mature version known as dry onions. The yellow onion with its pale colored skin, strong taste and white flesh is the most common variety. Red onions are a more mild variety with purple toned skin and reddish flesh. Green onions are characterized by their long green leaves and underdeveloped bulb. They are typically used in salads and soups.

To gain maximum health benefits, it is best to remove as little of the edible portion of the flesh as possible when removing the topmost, layer. The layers immediately below the brown paper layer contain the maximum nutrients and even removing tiny amounts of extra flesh can lead to a loss of significant amounts of its vital nutrients.

Minty Sweet Onion Juice Ingredients:

- 1 small onion
- A handful of fresh mint leaves
- 3 large carrots

Add-ons

- Celery
- Cucumber

Puree all ingredients until smooth, pour in tall glasses and enjoy.

Nutritional Information

A one cup serving of onions, is very low in sodium, and contains not fat or cholesterol. It contains only 48 calories and delivers a significant amount of fiber. They contain more polyphenols than garlic, tomatoes, leeks and carrots. Onions juice also contains ample amounts of vitamin C, B6, and folic acid along with minerals like calcium, iron, phosphorus, chromium and magnesium. The trace amounts of sulfur found in onions are accredited with many health benefits.

Health Benefits of onions

The variety of sulfur compounds housed in onions counter the effects of a number of cancers like esophageal, breast, renal, laryngeal and prostate. Sulfur is also one of the vital hair growth compounds.

When consumed on a regular basis onions lower cholesterol levels as well as the level of homocysteine, a possible cardiac stroke risk factor. Quercetin is a natural antihistamine found in onions that averts symptoms of allergies and asthma. Clinical studies show that the compound allyl propyl disulfide brings down blood sugar levels while the chromium aids in improving glucose tolerance. The dietary fiber, inulin aids digestion and is a food source for healthy bacteria. Consumption of raw onions is recommended for averting colds while its oils help to dissolve mucus.

The antibacterial properties of onions help in preventing tooth decay. According to research chewing on raw onions for a few minutes kills all germs in the mouth. A drop of onion juice eliminates ear aches, and used as a dressing diminishes boils, wounds and bruises.

Orange: Orange Smoothie

Full of natural sweetness and free from saturated fats, cholesterol and sodium, oranges provide an abundance of healthy nutrients. They are equally good when juiced with other fruits of choice or on their own.

Originating thousands of years ago in southern Asia, oranges are the largest citrus crop, and one of the most readily recognized fruit on the planet. Orange is the world's third most loved flavor following chocolate and vanilla. Oranges are in reality modified berries with pits holding volatile oil glands. The edible pulpy flesh is composed of carpels containing fluid-filled vesicles. The vesicles are nothing more than specialized hair cells. The soft, juicy orange pulp is enclosed in a bright orange outer rind.

Orange Smoothie Ingredients:

- 1 large orange peeled and segmented
- ¼ cup orange flavored yogurt
- 1 tsp. honey
- 4-5 ice cubes

Add the orange pieces into a blender and blend for about fifteen seconds. Then add the remaining ingredients and whiz for another 10 to 15 seconds to obtain a smooth drink. Pour into tall glasses and enjoy.

Add-ons

- Banana
- Coconut or almond milk

Nutritional Information

Compared to most other fruits and vegetables, oranges deliver more fiber. One medium sized orange also yields one gram of protein and only 80 calories. A single orange contains more than 170 varying phytochemicals and over 60 flavonoids. A large number of these compounds are known to provide anti-inflammatory, and antioxidant benefits.

One medium sized orange also supplies 93% of the daily recommended allowance of vitamin C, almost 10% folate, 9% vitamin B1, close to 7% potassium, copper and pantothenic acid and 5% calcium.

Health Benefits of Orange

The high vitamin C content in oranges helps to build immunity which fights infections and diseases. In combination with the antioxidants, vitamin C also hinders the process of aging by helping the formation of Callogen which eliminates wrinkles and keeps skin looking young. The elevated amount of fiber in the fruit is known to bring down blood glucose levels in people with type 2 diabetes and may improve insulin levels in people with type one diabetes.

The compound liminoid in oranges is linked with averting cancers of skin, lung, mouth, stomach and breast. Choline is another compound found in ample amounts in oranges, it aids muscle motion, sleep, transmission of nerve impulses and memory, in addition to helping with absorption of fat. Zeaxanthin and various carotenoids found in oranges have an adverse effect on cancer in general and prostate cancer specifically.

Papaya: Heavenly Papaya Smoothie

Called the "fruit of the angles" by Christopher Columbus, this once exotic fruit is loved all over the world for its nutritional, digestive and medicinal properties.

Also called the pawpaw or mamao fruit, there are two basic varieties of papayas available. The more common Hawaiian variety tends to be smaller in size, weighing on average one pound while the Mexican variety can weigh as much as 20 pounds. The Hawaiian variety has a more intense flavor, but both tend to be delicious.

The skin of the fruit can range in colour from green to yellow-orange depending on the degree of ripeness. Fruit ready to eat will give way when pressed gently. The flesh is bright orange with a hollow centre containing peppercorn style seeds. The seeds are edible and held in high regard in traditional medicine due to their curative properties. The flesh has a sweet creamy taste with mild aroma.

Heavenly Papaya Smoothie Ingredients:

- 1 cup diced and frozen papaya
- ¼ plain yogurt
- ½ almond milk
- 4-5 large strawberries

Blend all ingredients in a blender for 30 – 40 seconds, or until a desired consistency is reached and enjoy!

Add-ons

- Chia Seeds
- Cinnamon

Nutritional Information

This tropical goldmine is loaded with nutrients. A one cup serving of 140 grams supplies 144% of the daily vitamin C requirements. It also supplies 31% of the day's vitamin A needs, 10% of the potassium needs, 4% of magnesium, 3% of each calcium, thiamin, riboflavin and pantothenic acid, 2% of niacin, and 1% of each iron, vitamin B6, phosphorus, zinc and copper. The story does not end here. The same serving also delivers one gram of protein and three grams of dietary fiber and only 55 calories. All this with the added benefit of no saturated fats, cholesterol and only trace amounts of sodium. Furthermore, papayas contain a number of very beneficial phytonutrients like alpha and beta carotene, zeaxanthin, lutein and lycopene.

Health Benefits of Papaya

Papayas house a number of exceptional enzymes including papain and chymopapain which have been linked with lowering inflammation and aiding against diseases like osteoarthritis and asthma. Additionally they aid in healing burns. The fiber in papaya is believed to bind to cancer-causing toxins in the colon and keeping it healthy. The flavonoids in papaya protect against lung and other cancers, while the antioxidants in the fruit delay the aging process by offering the body a large number of free radical scavengers.

The lack of cholesterol and elevated amounts of fiber aid in keeping cholesterol levels in check; the special digestive enzymes aid digestion by facilitating protein breakdown. The high water content of the fruit maintains regular bowel movements and prevents constipation.

Parsley: Green Parsley Smoothie

Parsley is a perennial plant known for its exceptional content of flavonoids and antioxidants which afford it some amazing disease preventing capabilities. It also adds a good flavor to numerous dishes.

Parsley has been cultivated for more than 2000 years as a medicinal plant as well as a culinary herb. The biennial plant develops into to beautiful foliage that is easy to grow and makes an ideal kitchen plant. Two basic varieties of the herb exist, curly leaf parsley named due to the ruffled look of the leaves and flat leaf parsley with more level leaves. The flat leaf parsley, also known as Italian parsley, has stronger aroma and is not as bitter as the curly leaf variety. Most commonly seen as nothing more than a decoration on a plate, parsley is actually a highly nutritious food.

Green Parsley Extract Ingredients:

- 1 cup chopped parsley
- 1 small cucumber
- 1 green apple
- 1 lemon
- 1teaspoon honey
- ½ cup of orange juice

Chop the apple an cucumber into pieces that the blender will handle with ease. Add the orange juice into a blender and add half of the parsley and blend until smooth and liquid. Add all other ingredients one by one, blending half a minute after each ingredient. Finally add the remaining parsley until silky smooth.

Add-ons

- Ginger

- Banana

Nutritional Information

Parsley is a total protein; meaning it houses all of the essential amino acids, 2 grams of protein and 2 grams of fiber in every fresh cup full and only around 22 calories. Parsley is a good source of a variety of minerals. One cup contains approximately 8% or 83 milligrams of calcium, 3.7 milligrams of iron, and it delivers ten per cent of the daily copper needs, seven per cent of magnesium and potassium needs, six per cent zinc and five per cent phosphorus.

Parsley is also a powerhouse of vitamins. Just one cup supplies 820% of the daily vitamin K requirement, 23% of folates, 89% of vitamin C in addition to 168% of vitamin A requirements.

Health Benefits of Parsley

Traditionally parsley has been useful in three main areas as a medicine. It is a diuretic and aids in removing excess water from the body, making it useful in offering relief from premenstrual water retention. It also aids flatulence that is brought on by colic pain. Parsley dressings are beneficial in relieving breast tenderness in lactating women. Rubbing parsley helps to soothe insect bites and heal bruises. Lastly parsley is recommended as prevention and breaking up kidney stones by the German Commission, an advisory panel of the government.

More recent research shows that a phytochemical found in the herb offers chemo-preventive properties. One study published in the Journal of Nutrition and Cancer found that people with greater parsley consumption had lower rates of lung cancer. The ample amounts of antioxidants protect against an array of diseases.

Peach: Filling Peach Smoothie

Traditionally peach trees were considered to be the trees of life. This is not surprising, considering they produce fruit that has truckloads of healthy nutrients to deliver.

By nature, peaches are a fuzzy fruit originating in China. A typical piece of the fruit resembles an apple and ranges from 7 to 10 cm in diameter. On average it weighs approximately 130 grams. There are two main varieties of the fruit, freestone and clingstone. The freestone variety refers to the variety in which the flesh can be easily separated from the pit by simply cutting the fruit in half and twisting the two halves in opposite directions. With the clingstone variety, the flesh sticks to the pit and cannot be separated from it entirely. In both varieties the flesh of the fruit can range in colour from orange-yellow to white, with white fleshed ones being sweeter and less acidic.

Filling Peach Smoothie Ingredients:

- 1 peach cut up with pits removed
- 4 tbsp rolled oats
- 1 banana frozen
- ½ cup almond milk
- Honey to taste

Add the oats to the almond milk and allow them to soak for about ten minutes. This allows oats to become soft. Place all ingredients in a blender and blend until smooth. Serve immediately.

Add-ons

- Chia seeds
- Fresh orange juice

Nutritional Information

The main attraction of peaches lies in the fact that they contain ten different kinds of vitamins along with a host of other nutrients. This includes vitamin A, C, E, K, B1 (thiamine), B2 (riboflavin), B3 (niacin), B5 (pantothenic acid), B6, and B9 (folate). It also contains trace amounts of a number of minerals that include calcium, iron, magnesium, manganese, phosphorus, potassium, sodium and zinc. Lastly peaches contain some important phytonutrients like Carotene-B, Crypto-xantin, and Leutein-zeaxanthin.

Health Benefits of Peaches

According to Texas AgriLife Research studies phenolic compounds in peaches offer anti-inflammatory, anti-obesity and anti-diabetic properties. These compounds may also potentially reduce the LDL (bad) cholesterol linked with heart diseases. The phenolic compounds which include anthocyanins, chlorogenic acids, quercetins and catechins all work collectively to fight off these diseases.

The ample amount of vitamin C in peaches is a potent antioxidant that helps to fight against the formation of free radicals that are known to lead to cancer. Additionally vitamin C aids in keeping the skin young looking by eliminating wrinkles. Peaches are also good for the digestive system. Their fiber and alkaline content prevents stomach ailments like constipation and irregular bowel movements.

Pear: Pearly Pear Juice

Homer described pears as the "gift of the gods" and this is not without reason. Pear juice is delicious on its own or combined with other fruits and vegetables. It is mild enough to be introduced to infants yet full of vital nutrients, fiber and antioxidants.

Pears are one of the oldest cultivated fruits on the planet. Roughly the size of an apple and skin that is paper thin ranging in colors from yellow to red, brown and green. Pears possess light colored flesh that is a bit grainy with juicy, sweet taste. Typically pears are bell-shaped, but more rounded varieties are also available.

A unique feature of pears is that they ripen best once picked. Commercial growers usually pick the mature fruit that is usually not yet ripe. Allowing them to sit on the kitchen counter for a day or two allows them to ripen fully. In order to speed up the process they may be left inside a brown paper bag. Pears begin to ripen from the inside, so to see if they are ready for consumption, gently press near the stem, if it is soft to the touch the fruit is ready. When the pear is soft to the touch around the middle, it is already overripe!

Pearly Pear Juice Ingredients:

- 2 firm pears
- 1 cup pineapple pieces
- 1 cm piece of fresh ginger
- 3-4 Ice cubes

Add-ons

- Green apples
- spinach

Nutritional Information

Pears are exceptional providers of water-soluble fiber, with one medium sized piece (about 160 grams) delivering roughly 20 per cent of the daily recommended allowance. They contain no sodium, saturated fat, or cholesterol and only 100 calories in addition to one gram of protein. They are also a good source of vitamin C, K, folate, iron copper, potassium and magnesium and contain a number of important phytochemicals like beta-carotene, lutein and zea-xanthin.

Health Benefits of Pears

The elevated amount of fiber in pears is beneficial for the heart. Studies show that fiber plays a key role in reducing bad cholesterol levels by binding it with bile salts and removing it from the body. Consumption of pears is associated with a reduction in the risk of stroke and being hypoallergenic it is safe for individuals who tend to develop allergic response with other fruits.

A Cornell University study found that the elevated antioxidant content of pears can help prevent brain related problems like Alzheimer's. The variety of vitamins like C and K and phytonutrients help to maintain the immune system and offer antioxidant as well as anti-inflammatory benefits.

Pineapple: Pineapple & Beetroot Juice

A native of South America, pineapple is a low calorie food with an array of unique health endorsing components. Once a rarity that only adorned the tables of royalty, it is now easily accessible for all to enjoy.

The pineapple is a fusion of many smaller fruits merged together around an inner core. This inner core serves a supporting function. The pulp of the fruit is fleshy and juicy with a sweet mildly tart flavor. The color of the ripe fruit ranges from yellowish to a reddish tone.

Once picked, the fruit does not ripen further, so it is best to seek out a piece that is heavy for its size to ensure that you get the best tasting one. While pineapples can be stored at room temperature, they do spoil easily, so it is best not to let them sit out for more than a day or two. Alternately, for the sake of convenience, the fruit can be cut, packaged and placed in the refrigerator soon after purchase. According to one study in the Journal of Agricultural and Food Chemistry this will not adversely affect its nutritional profile to any significant degree for six to nine days.

Pineapple & Beetroot Juice Ingredients:

- 2 cups fresh pineapple chunks
- One small beetroot
- Half a lemon
- Pinch of salt

Skin and core the pineapple and cut into small pieces. Wash the beetroot and cut into pieces after peeling.

Juice and serve.

Add-ons

- Cucumber

Nutritional Information

Pineapple is unique because it is the only known source of an enzyme called bromelain. It also supplies key nutrients like thiamin, vitamin A, C and B6, riboflavin, folate, pantothenic acid, magnesium, potassium, manganese, beta-carotene, polyphenols, calcium and iron. In fact one cup of freshly cut pineapple contains no fat or cholesterol, one gram of protein and 2.3 grams of fiber. All this goodness is accompanied with only a modest 83 calories per cup.

Health Benefits of Pineapple

The bromelain in pineapples is effective against a number of ailments. It is usefull in preventing blood clots and thus reduces the risk of heart attacks. Bromelain is also marketed in Germany as a natural anti-inflammatory supplement that may be effective against painful joints and is approved by Commission E. Being a digestive enzyme it is helpful against conditions like irritable bowel syndrome, gas and bloating.

The large amount of manganese in pineapples is beneficial for building healthy bones and strengthening weak ones. The beta-carotene is beneficial for good eyesight and reducing the risks of age related macular degradation. Furthermore, it has proven to play a positive role in deterring prostate cancer according to a Harvard School of Public Health's Department of Nutrition and hinder colon cancer in Japanese population.

Radish: Radish-Apple Juice

Radishes don't generally rank very high on most people's list of high priority vegetables, but this little nugget delivers a goldmine of health benefits and nutrients.

Radishes have been cherished since before the Roman Empire both as a food source and a medicinal product. They are a hardy plant frequently grown in combination with other plants due to their ability to draw pests away from the more sensitive plants.

Radishes can be grouped into for basic group types: summer, fall, winter and spring variety. Depending on the variety their size, shapes and colors also vary. Colors vary from red, pink, yellow, to white, while shapes range from round to elongated while size can range from small marble sized to some that are larger than a parsnip.

Radish-Apple Juice Ingredients:

- 4 medium sized radishes
- 1 apple
- 1 carrot
- 1 lemon
- Sea salt to taste

Wash all vegetables thoroughly. Cut so the fit the juicer with ease. Juice all ingredients and pour into glass.

Add-ons

- Cilantro
- Pear

Nutritional Information

Radishes have a very high water content (approximately 90%), which makes them great for anyone on a diet; but more than that they have almost no saturated fats, very little sugar and carbohydrates, and plenty of fiber. While many people toss radishes in salads, what they don't realize is that juicing them allows for faster delivery of all the nutrients they have to offer.

Radishes are a good source of potassium, vitamin C, folate, manganese, copper, magnesium, calcium, vitamin B6, riboflavin and sodium.

Health Benefits of Radishes

Radishes are excellent detoxifiers, helping to remove a large variety of toxins from different parts of the body. They aid digestion by regulating the flow of bile and bilirubin. Radishes are useful in controlling jaundice as they help to remove excess bilirubin from the liver. Regular consumption of radish juice can reduce inflammation of the urinary tract and prevent kidney infections. Furthermore radishes are known to help treat respiratory problems like asthma and bronchitis as they help to loosen mucus from the lungs. Recent studies show that radish juice can help to avert a number of cancers like stomach, colon, intestinal and kidney. The anthocyanins and vitamin C in the vegetable also inhibit the proliferation of cancerous cells.

Raspberries: Exotic Mango-Raspberry Smoothie

The addition of raspberries to your diet means acquiring the benefit of a wide range of nutrients. Furthermore the delicate, juicy fruit also delivers innumerable health benefits.

There are more than 200 species of raspberries, but the commercially grown varieties can be groped into three main groups: red, black and purple raspberries. They are known as an aggregate fruit, which means that they are a combination of numerous small individual fruits, each with its own seed. Raspberries have a generally tart taste but can be sweet as well. They are a great flavour enhancer in green smoothies, and absolutely delicious when combined with other fruits, yoghurt or milk.

Since raspberries have a short shelf life, it is best to use them within a day or two of purchase. The good news is that for longer storage, they can be frozen easily for up to a year without any loss of antioxidant activity. So stock up when they are in season and relatively inexpensive for year round use.

Exotic Mango-Raspberry Smoothie Ingredients:

- 1 cup raspberries
- 1 cup mango pieces
- 1 ½ cups chopped spinach
- ½ inch piece of fresh ginger
- 4-5 cubes of ice

Add-ons

- Kale
- Honey

Nutritional Information

One cup of fresh raspberries supplies 1.5 grams of protein, 8 grams of dietary fiber (which satisfies approximately 1/3 of the daily adult needs), and almost 15 grams of carbohydrates with a modest 64 calories. There is no shortage of vitamins and minerals in the fruit either. One cup also delivers 186 mg of potassium, 167 mcg of important carotenoids lutein and zeaxanthin, 31 mg of calcium, 111mg of copper, and 0.82 mg of manganese. Additionally it contains 9.6 micrograms of vitamin K, 32 milligrams of vitamin C and26 mcg of folate.

Health Benefits of Raspberries

Raspberries contain some powerful antioxidants which are responsible for slowing down the ageing process through neutralization of free radicals. The same flavonoids that afford raspberries their red color also stimulate the production of collagen and delay wrinkles. These phytonutrients, particularly anthocyanins also provide antimicrobial protection while ellagic and gallic acids offer protection against cancer.

The high fiber content of raspberries helps you to feel full longer and combined with their low caloric content means they can help with any weight loss program. Fiber is also known to lower cholesterol thus maintaining cardiovascular health. Lastly, fiber plays a vital role in maintaining regular bowel movements.

Spinach: Green Spinach Smoothie

Juicing spinach or consuming it in a smoothie is one of the best ways to benefit from its purifying and cleansing properties. To ensure maximum absorption of valuable nutrients like iron combine it with fruits and vegetables having high vitamin C content like tomatoes or oranges.

For juicing and smoothie preparations, it is best to choose fresh baby spinach leaves as they are tender as opposed the mature leaves which may be stringy or leathery. Freezing the leaves weakens the health benefits, while cooking for just two minutes enhances the benefits. Only half a cup of cooked spinach delivers three times as many nutrients as one cup of the raw vegetable! Hence, steaming the leaves in minimum amount of water for two minutes, then using the mixture in drinks provides maximum benefits.

Green Spinach Smoothie Ingredients:

- ½ cup freshly steamed, then cooled to room temperature spinach
- ½ cup pineapple juice
- 1 cup frozen strawberries
- 3-4 ice cubes

Blend all ingredients together until smooth, add ice and enjoy.

Add-ons

- Ginger
- Carrot

Nutritional Information

Spinach is one of the richest sources of iron with 100 grams supplying 25% of the daily recommended allowance. In addition, the same quantity satisfies nearly 47% of the daily needs of vitamin C, and 402% of the vitamin K needs. It also contains significant amounts of vitamin A, B6 (pyridoxine), B1 (thiamin), riboflavin, folates and niacin. Furthermore, it supplies good amounts of minerals like manganese, magnesium, potassium, zinc and copper, along with antioxidant phytonutrients like, beta-carotene, lutein, zea-zanthin and omega-3 fatty acids.

Health Benefits of Spinach

Spinach contains the antioxidant alpha-lipoic acid which has been shown to reduce glucose levels in the blood and enhance insulin sensitivity. Dark green leafed vegetables like spinach house chlorophyll which is successful against preventing cancerous effects of heterocyclic amines, compounds produced during high temperature grilling of foods. The high amounts of vitamin K in spinach aids calcium absorption, which leads to enhanced bone health. Deficiency of iron is a commonly associated with premature hair loss, which can be rectified with iron rich foods like spinach.

While everyone is familiar with bone building benefits of iron, not many people realize that it is also good for digestion. Spinach protects the lining of the stomach which prevents ulcers and eases constipation. Additionally it removes toxins from the colon. The abundance of nutrients in spinach like vitamin A are beneficial for growth of body tissues like skin while vitamin C is necessary for building collagen, a compound necessary for young looking skin.

Strawberries: Fast & Easy Strawberry Smoothie

Strawberries are known as the "queen of fruits" in Asian countries due to the health benefits they offer. When compared with other commonly grown fruits like bananas or apples, they deliver the greatest amount of nutrients.

Throughout the ages the strawberry has represented different things for different people. Due to its shape and colour, it was used as a symbol for Venus, the Goddess of Love. It represented perfection and righteousness to medieval stone masons which is why they carved in churches and cathedrals. The ancient Romans believed the fruit had tremendous medicinal value and they used it to treat a wide array of ailments.

More accurately known as a "false fruit", the juicy red strawberry is in reality a repository of the strawberry flower. In fact it is not even a true berry, because true berries have seeds on the inside and each strawberry has roughly 200 seeds scattered around the outside. Despite the oddities, strawberries are widely loved all over the world.

Fast & Easy Strawberry Smoothie Ingredients:

- 5-6 large strawberries
- ½ cup yogurt
- Honey to taste
- 4 or 5 large ice cube

Blend everything to a desired consistency and enjoy. If frozen strawberries are used, add half a cup of water instead of ice cubes.

Add-ons

- Bananas

Nutritional Information

Strawberries are loaded with nutritious vitamins, minerals and antioxidants. A 100 gram serving contains only 32 calories, 2 grams of dietary fiber, 91 grams of water, 7.7 grams of carbohydrates and 0.67 grams of protein. It contains negligible amount of fat and no cholesterol.

Among the vitamins it houses are vitamin A, C, B1, B2, B3, E, K and folate. It is also a potent source of minerals like calcium, magnesium, potassium, phosphorus, iron and zinc.

Health Benefits of Strawberry

Strawberries are full of antioxidants like anthocyanins and ellagitannins which are beneficial in reducing the risks of cardiovascular disease and cancer. Eating strawberries also helps to remove harmful substances from the blood. Additionally, they are good for averting inflammatory diseases like rheumatoid arthritis. Minerals like potassium and magnesium, which are found in abundant amounts in strawberries, are useful in reducing blood pressure. It is also believed that a number of compounds found in strawberries help to slow down the speed at which the brain ages, while the folates in the berries prevent birth defects.

The nitrates in strawberries have the potential of enhancing blood and oxygen flow to the muscles by seven per cent. This helps to minimize muscle fatigue, which means one can exercise for longer durations. According to tests, nitrate rich foods such as strawberries helped to burn more calories in dieting subjects, as opposed to those not eating strawberries.

Tomato: Satisfying Tomato Juice

Regardless of whether you call a tomato a fruit or a vegetable, the fact remains that this is one nutrient rich food that people should use more liberally.

The tomato is often described as a "functional food," implying that it delivers more than just the basic nutrients. Grown in every corner of the world, there are hundreds of tomato varieties available, 25,000 according to U.S. Department of Agriculture. They vary from each other on the basis of appearance, flavor and texture. Despite how the tomato is grown, organically or conventionally, there is little difference in the overall nutritional value. However, different varieties do have different antioxidant capacities.

Cooking tomatoes actually enhances their nutritional value. According to one 2002 study tomatoes cooked for thirty minutes increased the lycopene content by 35%. This is because heating breaks down the thick cell walls and releases the nutrients bound to them. Since tomatoes hold such an abundant supply of nutrients, it is not important whether you drink raw tomato juice or use a cook tomato juice recipe, as long as you do drink it.

Satisfying Tomato Juice Ingredients:

- 5 tomatoes
- 2 carrots
- 2 stalks of celery
- Salt & black pepper to taste

Thoroughly wash and cut all vegetables into pieces that your juicer can accommodate with ease. After juicing add the salt and pepper, and chill before serving.

Add-ons

- Juice of one lemon
- Mint leaves

Nutritional Information

One medium sized tomato delivers approximately 22 calories, one gram of fiber, one gram of protein, almost no fat or cholesterol, and five grams of carbohydrates. They contain a large variety of vitamins which include vitamin A, C, E, K and B6 in addition to thiamine, riboflavin, niacin, folate and pantothenic acid. Tomatoes are not in any way lacking in minerals either. They contain potassium, phosphorus, magnesium, calcium, sodium, iron, manganese, copper and zinc.

Tomatoes are best known however, for their ample quantities of antioxidants which include alpha-lipoic acid, lycopene, choline, folic acid, beta-carotene and lutein to name a few.

Health Benefits of Tomato

The antioxidants in tomatoes are beneficial for a wide range of ailments. The alpha-lipoic acid aids in converting glucose to energy and some evidence indicates that it can help control blood glucose levels. This in turn protects retinopathy in diabetic patients and perhaps even wards off nerve tissue and brain damage. The choline aids in reducing chronic inflammation which is linked to many chronic diseases like osteoporosis, cancer and cardiovascular diseases. The excessive amount of lycopene found in tomatoes is an exceptional scavenger of cancer causing free radicals. The Beta-carotene along with lycopene protects the skin from sun's UV light that leads to premature wrinkles.

Turmeric: Golden Tropical Turmeric Smoothie

Used for more than four thousand years as a food and medicine in the South Asian countries, the active ingredient in turmeric has the potential to ward off cancer and dementia.

Belonging to the same family as ginger, the turmeric plant is commonly cultivated in India, China and tropical Asia. The thick rhizome has brown skin similar to that found on ginger and is bright orange-yellow inside. The tubers are collected cleaned and dried for culinary purposes as well as medicinal use.

The deep-orange turmeric pigment has been employed as a dye since ancient times, and is a vital ingredient in Chinese as well as Ayuvedic medicines. Turmeric has also been held in high regard in Indian religious ceremonies for centuries. The National Center for Complementary and Alternative Medicine endorses curcumin, the active ingredient in turmeric, as a potential supplement based on preliminary evidence.

Golden Tropical Turmeric Smoothie Ingredients:

- 1 cup almond milk
- 1 cup mango chunks
- ½ teaspoon powdered turmeric
- Honey to taste (optional)

Blend everything until smooth and creamy and enjoy chilled.

Add-ons

- Pineapple
- Papaya

Nutritional Information

An initial view of turmeric's nutritional profile may not appear to be highly impressive. Two teaspoons of powdered turmeric contains 16 calories, elevated levels of magnesium (17% of the daily recommended dosage), and iron (10 % of the daily requirement.) Additionally it contains moderate amounts of vitamin B6, copper, potassium and fiber.

The nutrient of interest in turmeric however is curcumin, a strong anti-inflammatory agent that has attained significant attention recently due to its high potential as a cancer and Alzheimer preventing agent.

Health Benefits of Turmeric

According to laboratory and animal studies, turmeric and its primary constituent curcumin have been shown to possess antioxidant, anti-cancer and anti-inflammatory properties. Nutritionist Jonny Bowden, in his book states that numerous studies have shown curcumin to be successful in "either reducing the number or size of tumours or the percentage of animals who developed them." Furthermore, researchers believe that the compound's anti-inflammatory properties may have sufficient strength to break apart the amyloid plaques that play a vital part in Alzheimer's disease.

Initial studies also indicate that turmeric might be helpful in reducing the gravity of viral and bacterial infections. It may also aid in improving insulin sensitivity in diabetic patients, as in animal studies it caused sugar levels in the blood to drop.

Turnip: Appetizing Turnip Juice

The nutrients supplied by the juice of turnip root and its greens offer an ideal way for "powering up." The vegetable provides a large variety of essential vitamins, minerals and fiber.

Turnip roots have been used as a source food since the ancient Greek and Roman times. While it is the root that has always been the more desirable staple food, it is the top greens which are many times more potent in important antioxidants, vitamins and minerals.

Being conical to roundish in shape, the turnip flesh is typically white and at times contains streaks of pinkish, to purple streaks. Baby turnips, picked in early stages of growth, prior to reaching maturity, have a more delicate sweet flavor compared to the fully mature root. The mature root can reach weights of up to 1 kg, and has a more pungent flavor with firm and woody texture. Turnips are in season from fall through winter months.

Appetizing Turnip Juice Ingredients:

- 1 heaping cup of cubed turnips
- 1 cup cabbage
- 2 carrots cut up
- 1 apple cut up
- Handful of mint leaves

Wash all ingredients well and cut into size that will fit the juicer with ease. Juice all ingredients and enjoy.

Add-ons

- Turnip Greens

Nutritional Information

When it comes to nutrients, turnips contain a mindboggling list that is sure to impress even the most health conscious individuals. For juicing purposes, it is best to buy turnips with the greens intact as they contain more than a day's supply of some vital nutrients. A single cup serving of the fresh root contains only 28 calories and delivers 27 milligrams of vitamin C. This is more than 30% of the daily recommended allowance. In addition turnips supply vitamins B-2, B-3, B-9, E and K and the minerals magnesium, potassium, phosphorus and zinc.

Juicing turnip greens along with the root further enhances the nutritional value of the juice, adding significant amounts of nutrients like omega-3 fats, iron, vitamin A, folate, copper, calcium, selenium , manganese and antioxidants like lutein, and zeaxanthin in addition to alpha and beta carotenoids.

Health Benefits of Turnips

To gain maximum benefits of turnip juice is to combine it with vegetables that are high in magnesium which allow for maximum absorption of the calcium in turnip. Turnip juice is beneficial for skin issues like acne, in addition to alleviating bladder issues, arthritis and anemia. Combined with lemon juice, turnip juice can help to provide relief from colds and cough.

One study published in "International Journal of Oncology" in 2010 states that phytonutrients known as indoles found in turnips killed human colon cancer cells. Other phytonutrients known as glucosinolates also found in turnips offer protection against prostatic hypertrophy, an inflammation related condition that may be the forbearer of prostate cancer. Additionally, this sulfur-infused compound provides anti-parasitic, anti-bacterial and anti-fungal protection.

Watercress: Basic Watercress Drink

Oozing with vitamins and minerals, this little leaf with its peppery flavor, tops the list of natural super-foods. It has been used since ancient times as a flavoring, aphrodisiac and for medicinal purposes.

One of the earliest leaf vegetables used for human consumption, watercress is considered to be a weed in many regions of the world, but is also a prized herb or an aquatic vegetable in many other regions. The plant is composed of hollow stems that float and small round leaves arranged around a common axis. For best flavor the leaves have to be harvested before the flat clusters of white flowers known as corymbs appear. The flowers turn into pods containing a double row of seeds which upon reaching maturity are edible. After flowering the leaves however turn bitter and are no longer suitable for eating.

Basic Watercress Drink Ingredients:

- 1 cup chopped watercress (34 grams)
- 1 large green apple
- 1 lime juiced
- 1 large cucumber

Wash and chop the ingredients so they will fit the juicer with ease. Juice and enjoy!

Add-ons

- Celery
- Kiwi
- pear

Nutritional Information

Watercress is a highly nutritious vegetable/herb. In fact the Egyptian Pharoahs made it available to their slaves to improve productivity! One cup (34 grams), of the raw stuff contains only four calories and no sugar, carbohydrates or fats. Additionally it supplies one gram of protein and a small amount of dietary fiber.

Watercress is particularly rich in vitamins and minerals providing a wide array of the most vital nutrients. A single cup serving delivers 32% of the daily vitamin A supply, 24% of vitamin C, 106% of vitamin K and 2% of vitamin E. Furthermore, it supplies 1% of the folate requirements. Watercress is certainly not lacking in any way in the mineral department either. A single cup serving supplies 4% of the calcium and manganese needs, 3% of potassium, 2% of magnesium and phosphorus, and 1% sodium. Lastly, watercress is also good supplier of some important flavonoid antioxidants like lutein, carotene and zeaxanthin. It also contains elevated amounts of glucosinolate compounds.

Health Benefits of Watercress

According to the latest studies the glucosinolates in watercress have strong anti-cancer effects. Consumption of such compounds averts the formation of breast colon, lung and prostate cancers. The antioxidants in the vegetable avert age related vision problems and aid in protecting against damage caused to the healthy cells by free radicals.

The ample amounts of vitamin K promotes good bone health and also minimize damage to the neurons in the brain thus aiding against Alzheimer's disease. A wide range of phytochemicals found in watercress aid in maintaining healthy skin. In fact according to one study, a significant improvement in skin tone along with reduction in wrinkles was observed in almost all study participants after just four weeks of watercress consumption. An amazing 39% decrease in wrinkles was recorded in one of the study participants.

Watermelon: Cooling Watermelon Juice

Contrary to the common conviction that watermelon is nothing more than sugar and water, it is in reality a nutrient dense food. This means it is a food that delivers elevated quantities of minerals, vitamins and antioxidants at low calorie cost.

There are over 1200 varieties of watermelons grown in 96 countries of the world. Their shape varies from oval, to round and square, to make tacking easier while the flesh colour ranges from red to yellow. The newer varieties have been crossbred to deliver more frit and thinner rind.

A close relative of cucumbers, squash and pumpkins, the watermelon is a negative-calorie food. This means that the body has to burn more calories to digest the fruit than it provides. Better even is the fact that every part of the it is edible including seeds and rind. Most watermelons range in weight from five to fifty pounds, and due to their large size it is possible to purchase portions of the fruits in many grocery stores.

Cooling Watermelon Juice Ingredients

- 2 cups seeded watermelon cubes
- Handfull of mint leaves
- Juice of one lemon
- Salt to taste
- Honey (optional)

Add all ingredients in a blender and process at high speed for 30 to 40 seconds. Pour into a tall glass and enjoy.

Add-ons

- Ginger

- Mango
- strawberries

Nutritional Information

One cup of diced watermelon, approximately 150 grams delivers only 43 calories, no fat or cholesterol, and one gram of fiber. The same one cup serving fulfills 17% of the daily recommended allowance of vitamin A, 21% vitamin C, 2% iron and 1% calcium. Additionally, watermelons provide vitamin B-6, niacin, riboflavin, thiamin, folate, pantothenic acid, magnesium, potassium, copper, zinc, phosphorus, selenium, manganese, choline, lycopene and betaine. In fact watermelons house more of the vital nutrient lycopene than any other fruit or veggie.

Health Benefits of Watermelon

Considering that watermelons are roughly 92% water, they make for great hydrating drinks. One Journal of Agricultural Food and Chemistry study even found drinking watermelon juice before a workout to cut down on muscle soreness the day after the workout and reduce heart rates. This is accredited to the rich amino acid content of L-citrulline in watermelons which aid in relaxing blood vessels and improving circulation.

The antioxidant lycopene found in abundant quantities in the fruit, is believed to have the capacity to not only treat, but prevent prostate cancer. It is also linked with the prevention of cardiovascular disease. Furthermore, extracts of watermelon has been shown to reduce blood pressure in obese middle-aged patients and aid in improving arterial function according to a study published in the American Journal of Hypertension. Choline, another vital nutrient in watermelons is associated with improving nerve impulse transmission, maintaining cellular membrane structure as well as aid in sleep, muscle motion in addition to memory and learning.

Wheatgrass: Wheatgrass Tonic

Wheatgrass is an amazing food that is loaded with seventeen amino acids, the building blocks of proteins and 92 out of the 102 minerals found in nature. It is the miracle food that must be included in everyone's daily diet.

Wheatgrass is grown from the seed of the common wheat plant. The grass is harvested when it is at the peak of its nutritional value, at about the height of seven inches. At this point it contains the greatest concentration of minerals, vitamins, amino acids, living enzymes, antioxidants, chlorophyll and phytonutrients that are not available in the fully developed wheat plant.

Wheatgrass is thought to be by many a complete food due to its diverse nutritional profile. A large handful of the grass yields roughly one ounce of juice which may be consumed on its own or combined with other fruits or vegetables. While the grass can last a few days in the refrigerator, the juice is best used immediately.

Recipe Title Ingredients

- ½ cup of finely chopped wheatgrass
- 2 apples
- 1 cucumber
- Juice ½ a lemon

After washing the vegetables chop them into pieces small enough to fit the juicer and juice. Please note that a centrifugal juicer will not juice wheatgrass at all, you will need a masticating juicer or do it manually.

Add-ons

- Mint leaves

- Carrots

Nutritional Information

Wheatgrass is considered to be a complete food by many for a good reason. In addition to being loaded with some vital enzymes, phytonutrients and antioxidants it contains 17 amino acids, the stuff needed to build muscle tissue, and repair damaged cells. It also houses 92 out of the 102 naturally occurring minerals, the most important among which include calcium, iron, potassium, magnesium, zinc, copper, selenium and phosphorus. Ounce for ounce wheatgrass contains more vitamin C than oranges and roughly twice the amount of vitamin A as carrots! It is also an exceptional source of vitamins E, K in addition to Riboflavin, Thiamin, Niacin, Pantothenic Acid and vitamin B6.

Health Benefits of Wheatgrass

The variety of enzymes in wheatgrass offers a lot of benefits. The enzyme protease aids digestion, cytochrome oxidase is a known anti-oxidant, amylase facilitates digestion, trans-hydrogenase strengthens the heart muscles while superoxide dismutase, a component of all cells in the body is known to slow cellular aging, hence keeping you young longer.

Wheatgrass juice provides protection against toxins, cigarette smoke and heavy metal poisoning. In fact wheatgrass may even aid in dissolving scars that can form on lungs. Being a nutrient dense food it suppresses appetite thus helping weight loss in addition to stimulating metabolism.

What Next?

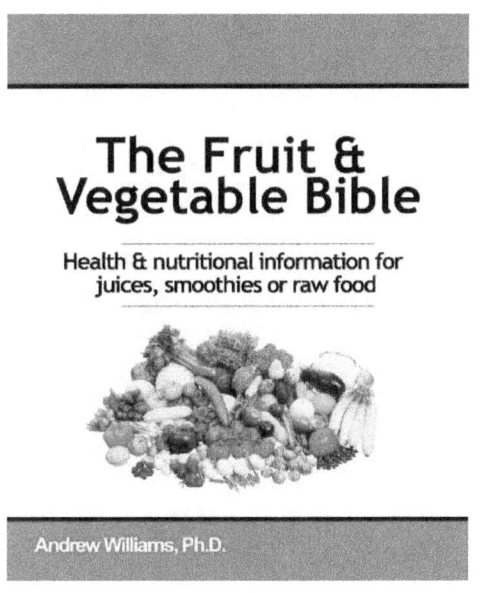

The Fruit & Vegetable Bible

Health & nutritional information for juices, smoothies or raw food

Andrew Williams, Ph.D.

If you enjoyed this book, why not pop over to my site, JuicingTheRainbow.com and introduce yourself. I'd love to hear from you.

You might also be interested in my Fruit & Vegetable Bible that contains a deeper analysis of the same 52 fruit, vegetables and herbs. It's available on Amazon in Kindle format and as a paperback. Search Amazon for it by name, or by its ASIN number, which is **B00JVPLDV0**.

You can also leave a review of this recipe book on Amazon if you want to help others find a better path to health and vitality.

Wishing you good health!

Andy Williams, Ph.D.